CLINICAL APPROACHES TO TACHYARRHYTHMIAS

edited by

A. John Camm, MD

Volume 8

CLINICAL APPROACHES TO TACHYARRHYTHMIAS
edited by

A. John Camm, MD
St. George's Hospital Medical School
London, United Kingdom

Volume 8

Ventricular Tachyarrhythmias in the Normal Heart
by

John P. Bourke, MD, FRCPI, FRCP (London)
Senior Lecturer in Cardiology
University of Newcastle upon Tyne
Consultant Cardiologist
Freeman Hospital
Newcastle upon Tyne, United Kingdom

and

J. Colin Doig, MB, FRCP (Glasgow)
Consultant Cardiologist
North Tyneside General Hospital
Newcastle upon Tyne, United Kingdom

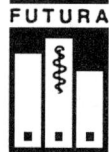

FUTURA

Futura Publishing Company, Inc.
Armonk, NY

Library of Congress Cataloging-in-Publication Data

for Library of Congress

CIP

Published by
Futura Publishing Company, Inc.
135 Bedford Road
Armonk, New York 10504-0418

ISBN #: 0-87993-400-X

Every effort has been made to ensure that the information in this book is as up to date and as accurate as possible at the time of publication. However, due to the constant developments in medicine, neither the author, nor the editor, nor the publisher can accept any legal or any other responsibility for any errors or omissions that may occur.

Printed in the United States of America.
This book is printed on acid-free paper.

Foreword

When all is said and done, cardiac tachyarrhythmias account for considerable distress and untimely death. The arrhythmias may only be a consequence of a more serious underlying pathology, but irrespective of its pathophysiology an arrhythmia may pose a serious risk or a difficult medical problem. Tachyarrhythmias must, therefore, be diagnosed and treated with great care and expertise.

For too long the cardiologist and the arrhythmologist/electrophysiologist have guarded their professional skills as secrets. In the past, the physician used the electrocardiogram and the electrophysiological study to establish accurate diagnoses, but the therapeutic consequences of these erudite diagnoses were negligible until the advent of electrophysiological surgery. Now the introduction of techniques of catheter ablation have catapulted cardiac electrophysiology into the medical headlines.

The mechanism of a cardiac arrhythmia is fundamentally important if therapy can be directed specifically toward that mechanism. Without knowledge of the target, the therapy cannot be aimed in the right direction. Some of our more successful therapies are "blunderbuss" treatments, such as amiodarone and the implantable cardioverter defibrillator. Irrespective of the cause of the arrhythmia, one of the many actions of amiodarone may well solve or suppress the problem. The cause of ventricular fibrillation is largely irrelevant to the corrective action taken by the implanted defibrillator. However, knowing, for example, that conduction through the right bundle branch is a critical component of bundle branch reentrant tachycardia, identifies an easy target for ablation therapy. Similarly, knowledge about the cellular mechanisms responsible for the long QT syndrome suggests obvious and specific antiarrhythmic medical and surgical approaches to the treatment. This specific approach to therapy, suggested recently in the *Sicilian Gambit*, must sometimes be at arm's length—applying assumptions from tissue or animal models to the human clinical situation. On the other hand, the much more detailed deductions that can now be drawn from the surface electrocardiogram and from intracardiac electrophysiological recordings allow the electrophysiologist to make measurements and experiments directly on the culprit arrhythmia. The effect of therapeutic interventions may then be easily reassessed and further therapeutic measures can be instituted until all is well.

The aim of this series of monographs, devoted to cardiac arrhythmology, is to update the physician and cardiologist and all of those responsible for caring for patients with cardiac arrhythmias about the spectacular developments in diagnostic and interventional cardiac electrophysiology. Hardly an arrhythmia fails to yield to the skills of the modern arrhythmologist. He/she no longer needs secrets; his/her successes are plain for all to see.

A. John Camm, M.D., Series Editor
Chairman of Medicine and Chief
Department of Cardiological Sciences
St. Georges's Hospital Medical School
London University
London, United Kingdom

Preface

Most ventricular tachyarrhythmias are associated with cardiac pathology; ischemic heart disease and cardiomyopathy are the most common causes. But some ventricular tachycardia (VT) occurs in patients who have no sign of any other heart disease. Unlike the VTs associated with heart disease, those occurring in normal hearts are rarely dangerous. There are two main varieties of "normal heart VT": right ventricular outflow tract tachycardia (RVOT) and fascicular tachycardia (FT). The mechanism of these tachycardias have still not been established, although microreentry, triggered activity, and automatic mechanism have all been thought responsible. The acquired forms of the long QT syndrome also occur in apparently normal hearts, although it is strongly suspected that underlying genetic ion channel abnormalities will soon be identified as their cause.

Both RVOT and FT are easily identified from the surface electrocardiogram because they generally have such classic appearances. RVOT is often described as similar to "left bundle branch block with right axis deviation" and FT most often resembles "left bundle branch block with right axis deviation (sometimes left axis deviation)." The benign form of RVOT must be distinguished from more sinister right VTs caused by arrhythmogenic right ventricular cardiomyopathy, diffuse cardiomyopathy, myocarditis, congenital heart disease and its surgery, etc. FT is often confused with supraventricular tachycardia because the QRS complexes are relatively narrow and resemble conducted beats, the tachycardia is often slow, and intervening baseline is often seen.

Usually these tachycardias are readily responsive to diverse therapies: sodium channel inhibitors, calcium antagonists, and β-blockers may all be effective. Adenosine will terminate some RVOT, and this result may cause confusion with supraventricular tachycardia. Similarly, FT is often very sensitive to calcium antagonists, which should not usually be considered for the treatment of VT.

Nowadays symptomatic RVOT or FT can be treated with use of direct ablation techniques that offer a seemingly permanent cure. It should be said, however, that follow-up after "successful" ablation is still short, and more time is needed to fully assess the value of the treatment.

It is frustrating and disappointing that such good therapies have been developed before the cause of these arrhythmias is established. However, our inquisitive nature prevents therapeutic success from stifling research into the mechanisms of these tachycardias.

These tachycardias are abundantly described and are associated with a rich and rewarding literature that continues to grow at a fast pace. In this volume of CATA (Clinical Approaches to Tachyarrhythmias) John Bourke and Colin Doig review these fascinating tachycardias.

A. John Camm, M.D.
Series Editor

Contents

xi

Acknowledgment

The University Department of Cardiology is generously supported by the British Heart Foundation, 14 Fitzharding Street, London W1H 4DH, United Kingdom. The authors are particularly grateful to Mrs. Sheila Jamieson and Ms. Clare Lawson for their secretarial help in the preparation of this book.

Introduction

The label *normal heart ventricular tachycardia* has been used increasingly in recent years to describe arrhythmias occurring in the absence of structural heart disease in a heterogenous group of patients.[1,2] Although it says more about what is not the cause of the arrhythmia than what is, if used uniformly, the term is clinically useful—at least until our knowledge of the underlying electrical abnormalities increases sufficiently to allow an etiologically based classification. The term also implies that structural heart disease has been comprehensively excluded and it is usually taken to infer a benign prognosis.[1-3]

Has the Term Any Clinical Value?

Originally, ventricular tachycardias occurring in otherwise normal hearts were considered rare curiosities in comparison with the frequency of life-threatening arrhythmias in postinfarct and cardiomyopathic patients. The term *normal heart ventricular tachycardia* was coined initially to describe what would otherwise have

1

been nothing more than a collection of isolated case reports. There were three main uses for the pooling of these syndromes: (1) it allowed amalgamation of clinical experiences of these patients based on the investigations used to exclude other causes of arrhythmia; (2) it allowed management based on previous experiences in similar patients defined under this category; and (3) over time, it facilitated understanding of the underlying arrhythmogenic mechanisms. Although predominantly of nuisance rather than life-threatening implication, the recognition that these arrhythmias were amenable to catheter ablation has increased awareness about them recently, so that the diagnosis is now made more frequently. The success of catheter ablation for most forms of ventricular arrhythmia in this category makes it the treatment of choice, whenever therapy is justified by symptoms. Whether the increase in the frequency of this diagnosis is merely the unveiling of a previously underdiagnosed entity, facilitated by the growth in invasive electrophysiology of recent years or, more intriguingly, a real increase in incidence of a previously rare condition remains speculative.

Arrhythmias Included Under the "Normal Heart" Classification

Normal heart ventricular tachycardia indicates that the arrhythmia is ventricular in origin, that both right and left ventricles are structurally normal without evidence of abnormal dilatation or hypertrophy, and that there are not clinically significant valvular or coronary artery diseases accounting for the arrhythmias (Table 1). However, ventricular arrhythmias associated with the

Table 1

'Normal Heart' Ventricular Tachyarrhythmias: Classification	
	Mechanism
Cyclic AMP-mediated VT ● Right ventricular outflow tract ● Left ventricular outflow tract	*Triggered automatic*
Idiopathic left ventricular VT **(Fascicular or Verapamil-sensitive)** ● posterior fascicular reentrant VT ● anterior fascicular reentrant VT	*Reentry*
Bundle Branch Reentrant VT ● Left bundle branch VT ● Right bundle branch VT ● Interfascicular VT	*Reentry*
Pediatric VT	*Various*
Idiopathic Ventricular Fibrillation ● Brugada syndrome (ST elevation V₁) ● Coronary spasm variants ● Trivial anatomical abnormalities	*Various*
Congenital Long QT Syndrome **Acquired Long QT Syndrome**	*EAD + DAD-related triggered activity*

VT = ventricular tachyarrhythmia; EAD = early afterdepolarizations; DAD = delayed afterdepolarizations.

congenital long QT syndrome and idiopathic ventricular fibrillation (including Brugada syndrome)[4] fall into a gray zone, legitimately fitting the label but, probably because of their seriousness, not normally considered part of this diagnostic category. Similarly, those due to temporary biochemical upset[5] and those occurring as part of a multisystem disease, such as systemic lupus erythematosus, or because of the proarrhythmic actions of other drug therapies (including acquired long QT syndrome) are probably best excluded. Whether ventricular tachyarrhythmias occurring in the context of what would otherwise be considered trivial cardiac pathology should be excluded from this group of conditions is uncertain at present, especially as the relevance of the abnormality of the arrhythmia is often speculative.

In all of these circumstances where the "normal heart" category seems to confuse rather than help, it is important to remember that the label is synonymous with *primary electrical disease*, or *idiopathic ventricular arrhythmias* and is intended only as a temporary classification until each arrhythmia subgroup is fully elucidated. At that stage all of these terms will become obsolete and can most usefully be abandoned, since each subtype will then be defined by its own etiology, arrhythmic mechanism, natural history, and optimum therapy.

This volume includes discussion of the following subgroups of arrhythmias:

1. Cyclic AMP-mediated ventricular tachycardia (eg, right and left ventricular outflow tract tachycardias)
2. Idiopathic left ventricular tachycardia (ie, fascicular tachycardia, verapamil-sensitive tachycardia)
3. Bundle branch reentrant tachycardia
4. Pediatric ventricular tachycardias
5. Idiopathic ventricular fibrillation (eg, Brugada syndrome)
6. Acquired long QT syndrome

The congenital long QT syndrome is not discussed in any detail in this volume simply because it is already the focus of a separate book in this series in its own right.[1a]

Incidence and Presentation of Normal Heart Ventricular Tachycardia

Although recognized for more than 50 years, normal heart ventricular tachycardia has traditionally been considered rare in the absence of structural heart disease. It accounts for less than 10% of referrals to an electrophysiology service.[1b,6] However, this is likely to represent only the more troublesome end of the spectrum, since many patients with asymptomatic, infrequent, or nonsustained forms may never seek medical attention and, furthermore, the condition tends to be benign even if untreated.[7,8] Genuine differences in the incidence of some these arrhythmias are recognized in different populations. For example, idiopathic left ventricular tachycardia (ie, fascicular tachycardia/verapamil-sensitive ventricular tachycardia) is reported more commonly in Oriental than in European series.[2,3]

Patients who present with sustained forms of ventricular tachycardia in the absence of structural heart disease are usually young; typically mean ages 20 to 30 years.[9-12] The typical presentation is with symptoms of paroxysmal palpitations, sometimes associated with dizziness or presyncope. Right ventricular outflow tract tachycardia predominantly affects females and there is often a history of arrhythmia precipitation by stress on exercise. Even patients incapable of sustained tachycardia can experience disabling dyspnea and presyncope on exercise due to frequent isolated monomorphic ectopy. The hemodynamic effects of atrial cannon waves may explain the severity of symptoms, which can be further compounded by anxiety, in these patients. In such highly symptomatic patients, catheter ablation may be indicated.[5]

In contrast to the benign long-term outlook for most patients with normal heart ventricular tachycardia, the presentation of idiopathic ventricular fibrillation with cardiac arrest or major self-terminating syncope identifies patients at high risk of sudden death. All such patients who survive are likely to present for medical attention and those who die usually undergo post mortem examination because of the unexpected nature of the event. Of 42 adult patients resuscitated from documented ventricular fibrillation in one series, 10 (24%) were found to have no identifiable structural abnormality or coronary artery disease.[13,14] Sudden death in previously well children is extremely rare.[15-18] In adults who die suddenly, post mortem examination identifies no cardiac pathology in approximately 15% of cases.[19,20] Despite the outward similarities in the mode of death in these patients without structural heart disease, post mortem examination cannot distinguish between idiopathic ventricular fibrillation, long QT or pre-excitation syndromes, or atrioventricular (AV) block.[21] The true incidence of the congenital long QT syndrome is unknown and is likely to remain so until the diagnosis can be based on genetic rather than electrocardiographic (ECG) testing.[22,23]

The acquired long QT syndrome, due to a wide range of drugs and other factors, is probably quite common, but outside of research studies, it is only likely to be identified in those who develop clinical arrhythmias.[24]

What Investigations Define the Heart as Structurally Normal?

Before defining the arrhythmias as occurring in a "normal heart," left and right ventricular dysfunction must be excluded, as must valvular and ischemic heart disease.[25,26] The implications for longer term management of missing underlying dilated cardiomyopathy, arrhythmogenic right ventricular "dysplasia," ischemic heart disease, or hypertrophic cardiomyopathy and misclassifying them as normal heart arrhythmias are self-evident.[1,6,27] The occurrence of sustained ventricular tachycardia in any of these other categories carries a poor prognosis and calls for a much more aggressive plan of antiarrhythmic management than that indicated for patients without structural heart disease.[28-30]

In addition to a detailed history and physical examination, a minimum range of additional investigations appropriate to the age of the patient are therefore required (Table 2).[31] These should include chest x-ray, 12-lead ECG, and transthoracic echocardiogram, as a minimum, to complete the noninvasive evaluation. Exercise testing is useful not just for excluding coronary artery disease, when relevant, but also for evaluating arrhythmia inducibility on exercise stress.[7,8,32] Exclusion of left and right ventricular dysfunction may require several types of assessment in order to provide a definitive answer. While obvious left or right ventricular dysfunction can be readily identified by cineangiography, radionuclide ventriculography, or transthoracic echocardiography, lesser degrees or more focal abnormalities may require the greater sensitivity of transesophageal echocardiography or cine magnetic resonance imaging (cine-MRI).[33-35] The ability of cine-MRI particularly to identify myocardial abnormalities at an earlier stage than other imaging techniques and to allow myocardial tissue characterization is likely to make it an essential test for excluding secondary causes of tachycardia in the future. However, at present the clinical relevance of some of the

Table 2

Testing to Exclude Structural Heart Disease in 'Normal Heart' VT[#]

Mandatory:[**]	12-lead ECG 24-hour ECG Chest x-ray (posteroanterior and lateral) Transthoracic echocardiogram Blood biochemistry and hematology Exercise stress test (Bruce protocol)
Recommended:	Electrophysiology testing Cineangiograms (right and left ventricles) Radionuclide ventriculography Cine magnetic resonance imaging Coronary angiography (as age appropriate) Signal-averaged ECG Blood toxicology (substance abuse; drug levels) Class I antiarrhythmic drug provocation (Brugada syndrome)
Optional (research):	Cardiac biopsy Ergonovine provocation during coronary arteriography[251] Heart rate variability (time ± frequency domain) MIBG-imaging (asymmetry of cardiac sympathetic innervation)

[#]Comprehensive history and physical examination assumed; [**]may require repeating at intervals during follow-up; MIBG = 123-meta-iodobenzylguanidine scanning of the heart.

minor abnormalities identified by MRI remains to be determined and the test is not a prerequisite for classification.

At some hospitals, cardiac biopsies are included routinely as part of the evaluation to exclude structural or inflammatory heart disease.[36,37] Abnormalities of cardiac autonomic innervation have been identified in some patients with idiopathic forms of ventricular tachycardia on the basis of abnormal QT/RR behavior and myocardial radionuclide imaging.[32,38]

During follow-up of patients with normal heart ventricular tachycardia, periodic reassessments are appropriate to distinguish those developing evidence of cardiomyopathy or systemic disease from those with "primary electrical disease." This is especially important in defining longer term prognosis for clinically recognizable subgroups. As a rule of thumb, structural heart disease is likely to underlie the occurrence of multiple arrhythmia morphologies. Whereas, in structurally normal hearts, tachycardias of left bundle branch morphology arise in the right ventricle and those of right bundle branch morphology, in the left.

Possible Mechanisms Underlying Normal Heart Ventricular Tachycardia

The common types of ventricular tachycardia, such as in patients following myocardial infarction, are readily understood in terms of classic reentry.[39,40] This mechanism is confirmed by their reproducibility of inductions by programmed stimulation and termination by critically timed extrastimuli at electrophysiology testing. In contrast, many forms of ventricular tachycardia occurring in the absence of structural heart disease are not explained by classic reentry.[6,41] In vitro studies suggest criteria that can be applied to intact human situations favoring automatic and triggered automatic mechanisms of arrhythmia. These include induction by short-long pacing sequences rather than by programmed stimulation with critically timed extrastimuli, a lack of relationship between stimulation coupling intervals and the initial cycle length of tachycardia, induction by exercise or isoprenaline infusion without extrastimuli, and their response to verapamil, adenosine, or β-blockade. It is relatively easy to establish that a mechanism other than reentry underlies a particular arrhythmia. It is usually impossible, however, to define the exact mechanism in the intact human heart.[41] As a result, ventricular arrhythmias of this type have been categorized by terms such as *catecholamine-sensitive, exercise-provokable, verapamil-responsive*,[42] and *adenosine-sensitive*[43] and by their anatomical site of origin: right ventricular outflow tract, left ventricular septal, left ventricular outflow tract, or left ventricular apical. This plethora of different terms is confusing but reflects the state of understanding of the arrhythmia at the time of the particular report. There is considerable overlap between "categories" defined in this way and, unless this is fully appreciated, it may impede the appropriate association of arrhythmias of similar mechanism just because, for example, they arise in different locations.

The following is an attempt to summarize the rather confusing literature on the diverse forms of ventricular tachyarrhythmias whose only common feature may be that they occur in what appears at present to be a structurally normal heart.

Cyclic AMP-Mediated Ventricular Tachycardia

These arrhythmias are probably due to a cyclic AMP-mediated, triggered, automatic mechanism related to catecholamine sensitivity rather than to pure reentry or automaticity.[11,44-48] They occur as a result of delayed afterdepolarizations and are therefore facilitated by isoprenaline[49] or abrupt reduction in vagal tone.[50] The triggering mechanism is probably a parasystolic focus incompletely protected from sinus rhythm and is maintained by triggered repetitive activity.[6]

Typically, a patient with this arrhythmia is female, aged 20 to 35, with symptoms of palpitations reproducibly occurring under conditions of stress or after exertion. The arrhythmia itself usually takes the form of frequent monomorphic ventricular ectopy or nonsustained or sustained monomorphic ventricular tachycardia. Sustained forms are invariably well tolerated hemodynamically and typically occur during the deceleration of sinus rate following exertion. Some patients with frequent monomorphic ectopy who never experience sustained arrhythmias, however, may complain of profound exercise intolerance due to symptoms of presyncope or breathlessness sufficient to justify therapy.[12]

It is unknown whether patients progress through stages of increasingly frequent ectopy to nonsustained and sustained forms of the same morphology arrhythmia over time. Even untreated, the prognosis is considered benign[1-3,5-14,25,26,44-48,51-55]; however, isolated reports of sudden deaths have been attributed to this arrhythmia.[56]

In Western electrophysiology units, cyclic AMP-mediated ventricular tachycardia is more common than idiopathic left ventricular tachycardia (fascicular/vera-pamil-sensitive) and its incidence may be increasing. Monomorphic ectopy is usually present on 24-hour Holter recordings during the waking hours and increased during periods of activity. At electrophysiology study, the arrhythmia is not inducible or terminable by programmed stimulation using drive cycles and critically timed extrastimuli. Nor is it induced by long-short burst pacing sequences. The frequency of isolated ectopy, longer nonsustained runs, and sustained ventricular tachycardia, all of the same morphology, can usually be produced by an isoprenaline infusion (5 to 10 μg/min). Typically, any spontaneous ectopy present before isoprenaline is suppressed as the sinus rate accelerates, only to reemerge as the sinus tachycardia decelerates from its peak level. When patients are recumbent and sedated, however, the arrhythmia may disappear and be noninducible.

This form of arrhythmia responds variably to β-adrenergic blockade and verapamil[57] but radiofrequency catheter ablation is now the treatment of choice if any therapy is required for symptoms.[44,45,51,58] Long-term antiarrhythmic drug therapy is no longer acceptable to the majority of these young patients because of either adverse effects or dissatisfaction with the need for long-term medication.

Right Ventricular Outflow Tract Tachycardia

The most common form of cyclic AMP-mediated tachycardia is that arising in the right ventricular outflow tract. It is characterized by repetitive monomorphic tachycardia with a left bundle branch block and inferior axis

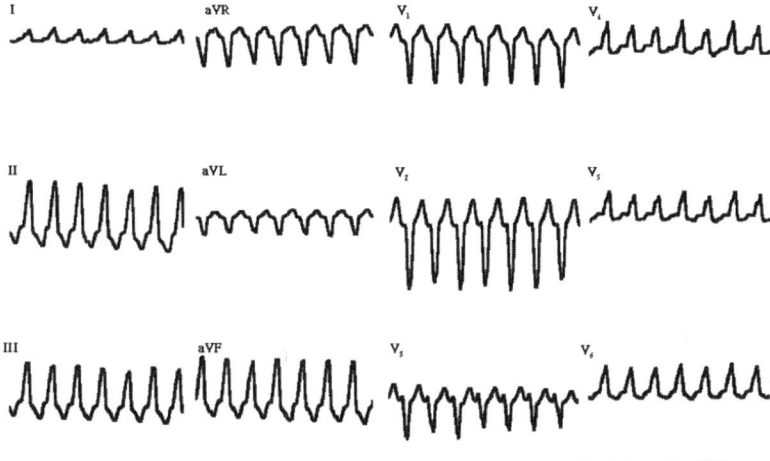

Figure 1. Right ventricular outflow tract tachycardia: 12-lead ECG. Note the left bundle branch block, inferior axis ECG morphology with negative complexes in V_1.

ECG pattern (Figure 1), occurring under the conditions described above.[51,59] Lead V_1 in tachycardia is negative in these patients. The main differential diagnosis is arrhythmogenic right ventricular dysplasia. In the normal heart group, however, there are no abnormalities in the right precordial ECG leads in sinus rhythm, no late potentials on signal-averaged ECG, and no fractionation of local electrograms at the site of origin of tachycardia in the right ventricular outflow tract in sinus rhythm (Figure 2).

The origin of the arrhythmia can be found by mapping spontaneous ectopy to find the site of earliest activation in the outflow tract (Figure 3). This is usually located just below the pulmonary valve on the septal or lateral aspect of the infundibulum (Figure 4).[60,61] Pace mapping at the site of earliest activation yields a 12-lead ECG identical to that of the spontaneous ectopic beats

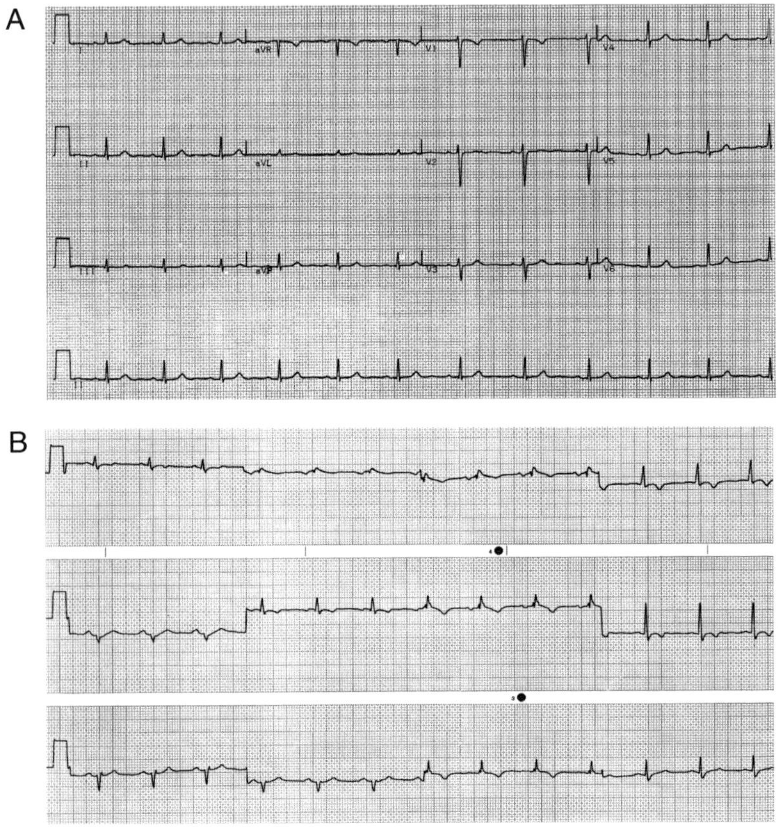

A

B

Figure 2. A. Right ventricular outflow tract tachycardia: normal SR ECG. **B.** Arrhythmogenic right ventricular dysplasia: abnormal SR EGC. Patients with arrhythmogenic right ventricular dysplasia usually have repolarization abnormalities in the right precordial leads or more extensively as in this example **(B)** on their 12-lead ECG in sinus rhythm (SR).

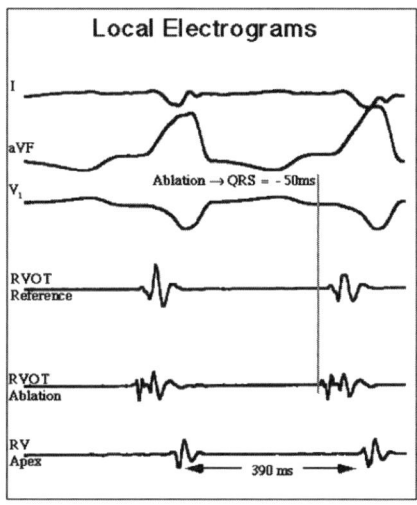

Figure 3. Local electrograms from right ventricular apex, outflow tract reference, and mapping catheter during sustained tachycardia. The local electrograms at the site of subsequent successful ablation times to 50 ms presurface QRS.

(Figure 5). The ready abolition of the arrhythmia within seconds of commencing energy delivery suggests that, in most cases, it arises in the immediately subendocardial cell layers, possibly from cells of the specialized conduction system in that region (Figure 6).[47] Success rates of ablation are of the order of 80% to 90% in reported series, but outcome depends primarily on the arrhythmia being present to guide activation mapping.[9,59,62-65] In patients whose arrhythmias are infrequent at the time of invasive testing, pace matching can be used to identify appropriate ablation sites; however, the success rate of such an approach is reduced. After successful ablation, there is no evidence to date that patients develop other foci of arrhythmia during follow-up. The main complication of concern during ablation is cardiac perforation

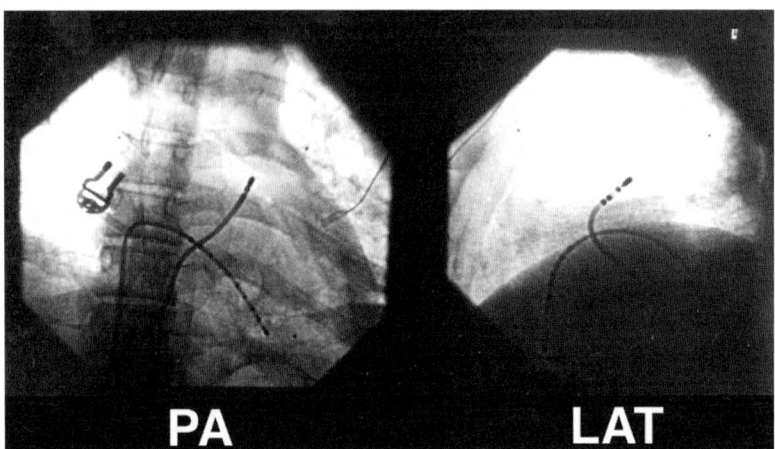

Figure 4. Right ventricular outflow tract tachycardia. Biplane—posterior and left lateral—projections of catheter at site of successful radiofrequency ablation, just below pulmonary valve. A decapolar reference catheter is situated in the right ventricular apex.

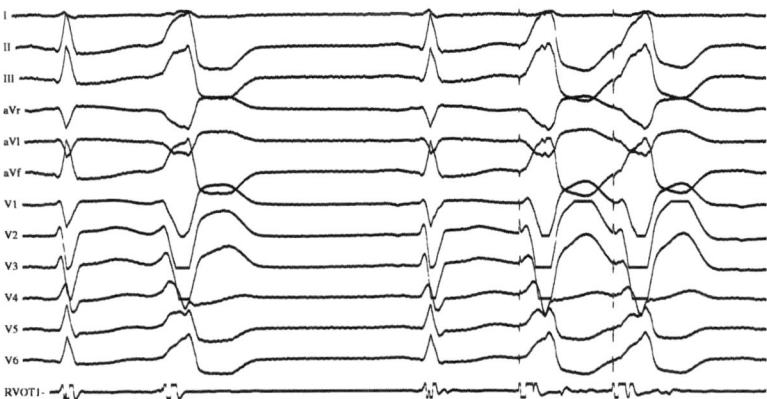

Figure 5. Right ventricular outflow tract tachycardia. Spontaneous ventricular ectopic beat from the right ventricular outflow tract is matched identically on all 12 leads of the standard ECG by pacing at the site of subsequent successful ablation.

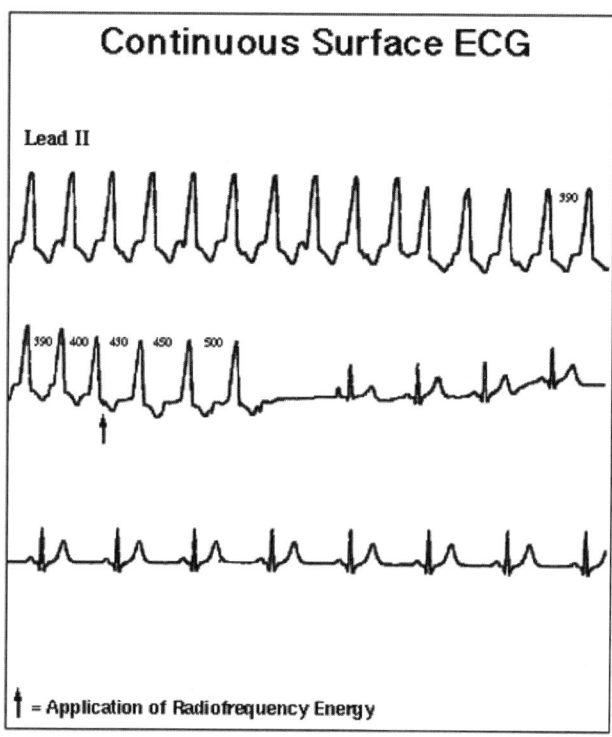

Figure 6. Right ventricular outflow tract tachycardia. Prompt abolition of sustained right ventricular outflow tract tachycardia by catheter ablation within five beats of commencing energy delivery. Note tachycardia cycle length increases progressively prior to termination.

with tamponade from burns in the thin-walled outflow tract.[52,66-68] It is more difficult to abolish the arrhythmia in some patients in whom a more extensive arrhythmogenic area has been described.[65] Although often discussed, there is little to support the view that these patients constitute part of the spectrum of arrhythmogenic right ventricular dysplasia and that they will go on to manifest progressive abnormalities. However, in this regard, the finding of structural abnormalities on MRI that resemble features of arrhythmogenic dysplasia in a substantial number of patients with idiopathic right ventricular outflow tract tachycardia despite normal right ventricular function and volume is of concern.[69] Therefore, until the relationship between these two conditions is better understood, it seems prudent to recommend periodic reassessments of right ventricular size and function even in patients who have undergone successful ablation of "idiopathic" tachycardia.

Repetitive Monomorphic Ventricular Tachycardia

Repetitive monomorphic ventricular tachycardia usually arises in the outflow tract of the right ventricle also, but unlike that described above, typically occurs at rest and is usually nonsustained. Its underlying mechanism is also cyclic AMP-mediated, and transient increases in sympathetic tone have been shown to occur before tachycardia initiation.[70,71] It is now postulated that right ventricular outflow tract tachycardias of both the exercise-induced and repetitive monomorphic nonsustained forms probably reflect disparate clinical manifestations of the same cyclic AMP-mediated triggered activity mechanism.[70,72] Therefore, there is now probably little value in classifying these two arrhythmias separately.

Left Ventricular Outflow Tract Tachycardia

Other morphologies of ventricular tachycardia have also been reported in patients whose arrhythmia behav-

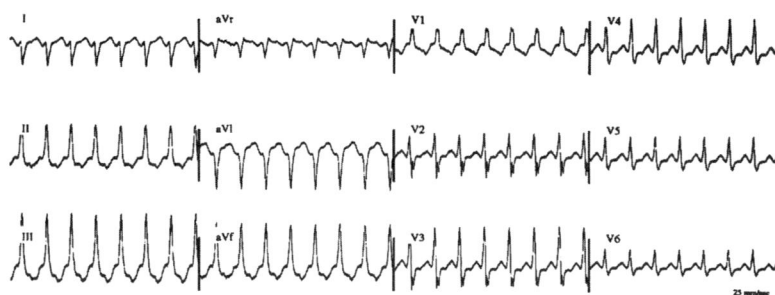

Figure 7. Left ventricular outflow tract tachycardia: 12-lead ECG. Note the right bundle branch inferior axis morphology distinguishing this from tachycardias of right ventricular outflow tract origin.

ior is compatible with a cyclic AMP-mediated triggered automatic mechanism.[9] The presence of a positive V_1 morphology in tachycardia suggests that the arrhythmia will not be ablatable from the right side of the heart (Figure 7). Some of these arrhythmias have been mapped to more epicardial sites in the outflow tract region close to the left main stem coronary artery.[73] Overenthusiastic attempts at ablation risk major infarction and are not justified at present.

In addition, however, there are isolated reports of arrhythmias with similar behavior that arise at sites in the left ventricle away from the septum and lower than the outflow tract.[47,48,54,55,74] Their importance is that they suggest that a type of arrhythmia, previously only associated with the right ventricle, can arise elsewhere. Three cases of idiopathic ventricular tachycardia reported by Sung et al[48] had features compatible with a cyclic AMP mechanism, although their site of origin within the left ventricle was not stated. Similar arrhythmia behavior from a posteroinferior left ventricular site in one patient was reported by Zipes et al[47] and from a left ventricular outflow tract site in two patients, by Lerman et al.[71] These latter cases are similar to the patient with left ventricular outflow tract illustrated here from the cardiology unit at Freeman Hospital (Figures 8 through 11). Combining the evidence from these various reports, it is probable that cyclic AMP-mediated tachycardia can arise from anywhere there is specialized conduction tissue partly insulated from sinus rhythm in either ventricle. It is the arrhythmia's behavior rather than its ECG morphology which suggests that it is likely to be amenable to catheter ablation. Although more common, right ventricular outflow tract tachycardia should no longer be viewed as a class by itself, defined by its site of origin; it should be viewed as a subclassification of arrhythmias with cyclic AMP-mediated mechanisms.

Idiopathic Left Ventricular Tachycardia (Verapamil-Sensitive/Fascicular)

Idiopathic left ventricular tachycardia presents typically in patients in the 20- to 30-year age group with palpitations due to sustained, relatively "narrow" QRS tachycardia. Two different ECG patterns of arrhythmia occur. The more common has right bundle branch block with left axis deviation and arises in the inferior septal region of the left ventricle (Figure 12). Less commonly the arrhythmia has complete right bundle branch block and right axis deviation and arises superior and superior-septally (Figure 13).[75,76] In the arrhythmia, QRS duration is usually less than 150 ms, which accounts for its frequent misdiagnosis as supraventricular tachycardia,[76-79] and the sinus rhythm ECG commonly shows transient

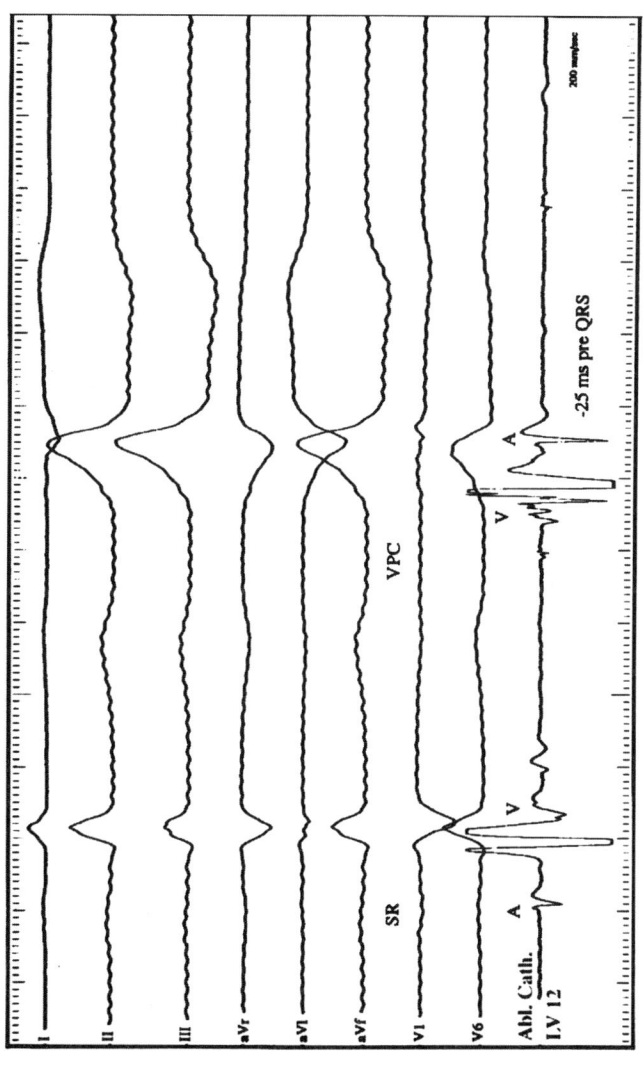

Figure 8. Left ventricular outflow tract tachycardia. Local electrogram timing in relation to QRS onset on the surface ECG of a sinus and an ectopic beat at the site of successful ablation before energy delivery. Note the atrial and ventricular components of the signal recorded, indicating the catheter's proximity to the atrioventricular ring.

30° RAO projection   60° LAO projection

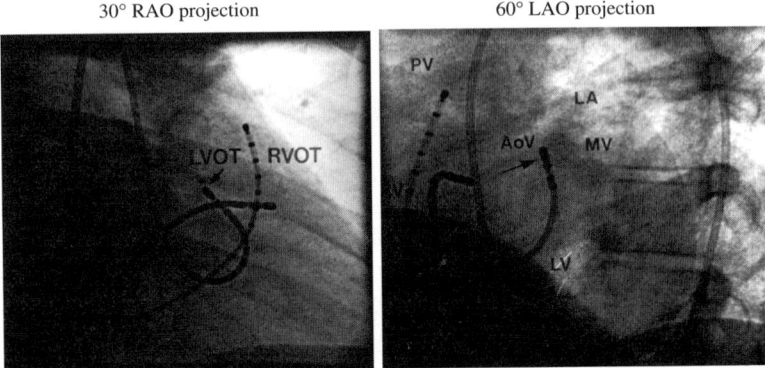

Figure 9. Cyclic AMP-mediated left ventricular outflow tract tachycardia. Polaris ablation catheter at the site of successful ablation of ventricular tachycardia in the left ventricular outflow tract (LVOT). The decapolar catheter is sited in the right ventricular outflow tract (RVOT) and the second Polaris catheter is in the His portion in the right ventricle. RAO = right anterior oblique; LAO = left anterior oblique; PV = pulmonary valve; AoV = aortic valve; LA = left atrium; RV = right ventricle; MV = mitral valve; LV = left ventricle.

inferolateral repolarization changes, particularly after tachycardia termination (Figure 14).[76] There is a male preponderance in most reported series and the incidence is lower in Europe and North America, for example, than in China and Japan. Most patients do not give a history of exercise or stress precipitation.

The prognosis in both forms of this arrhythmia is benign, although 16% of patients in one series had severely limiting symptoms and 46% had limiting symptoms that required therapy.[53,80] Cases of reversible tachycardia-induced cardiomyopathy have been reported, also emphasizing the potential dangers.[81]

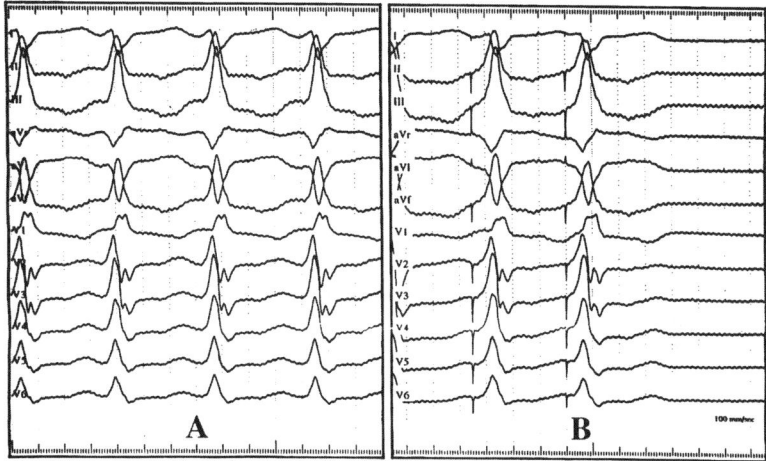

Figure 10. Left ventricular outflow tract tachycardia. Spontaneous ventricular tachycardia (**A**) arising in the left ventricular outflow tract is matched identically on all 12 leads of the standard ECG by pacing at the site of subsequent ablation.

Electrophysiology of Idiopathic Left Ventricular Tachycardia

Tachycardia is inducible in the majority of patients by use of critically timed ventricular extrastimuli. In these, there is an inverse relationship between the S_1S_2 and S_2VT coupling intervals at the initiation of tachycardia.[76,77,82] Induction is not usually facilitated by isoprenaline, and 1:1 ventriculoatrial conduction during tachycardia is common. Verapamil (5 to 10 mg i.v.) but not adenosine reliably terminates or profoundly slows tachycardia.[41,42,83-85] The intriguing finding in one patient of a site of localized fragmented activity near the posterior fascicle of the left bundle in sinus rhythm and continuous electrical activity at the same site during tachycardia

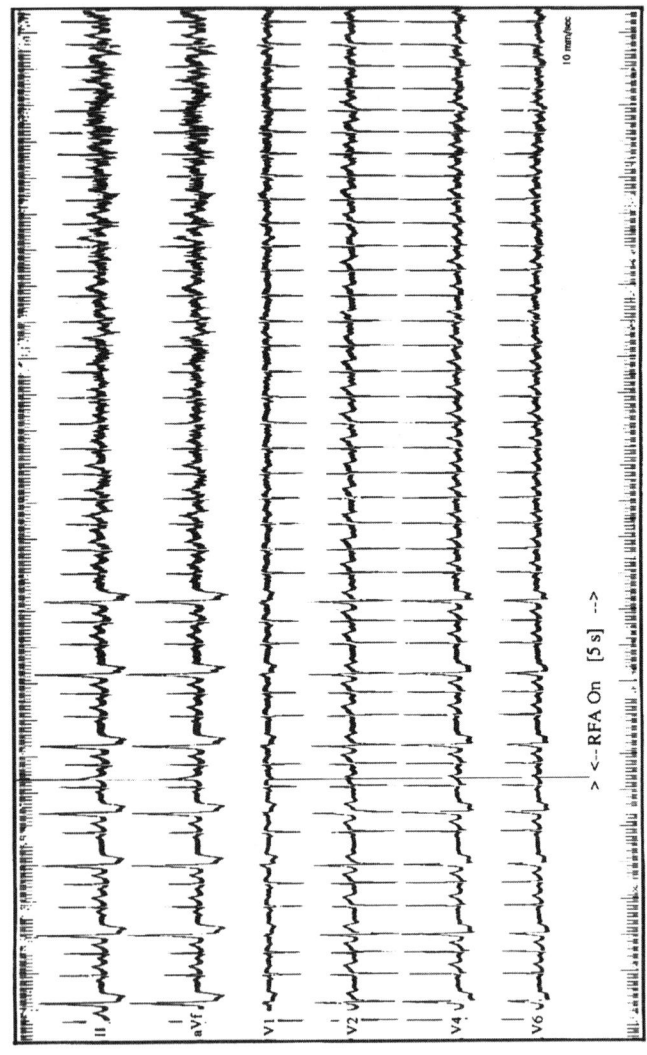

Figure 11. Left ventricular outflow tract tachycardia. Prompt abolition of left ventricular outflow tract ectopy by catheter ablation within 5 seconds of commencing energy delivery.

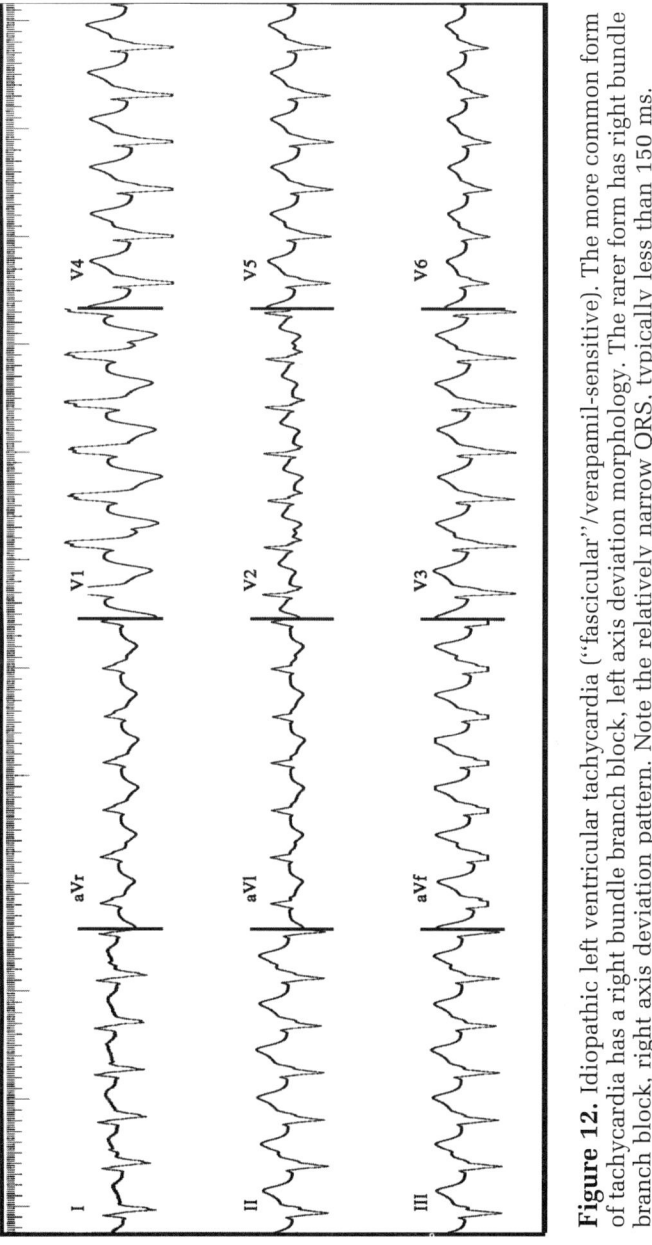

Figure 12. Idiopathic left ventricular tachycardia ("fascicular"/verapamil-sensitive). The more common form of tachycardia has a right bundle branch block, left axis deviation morphology. The rarer form has right bundle branch block, right axis deviation pattern. Note the relatively narrow QRS, typically less than 150 ms.

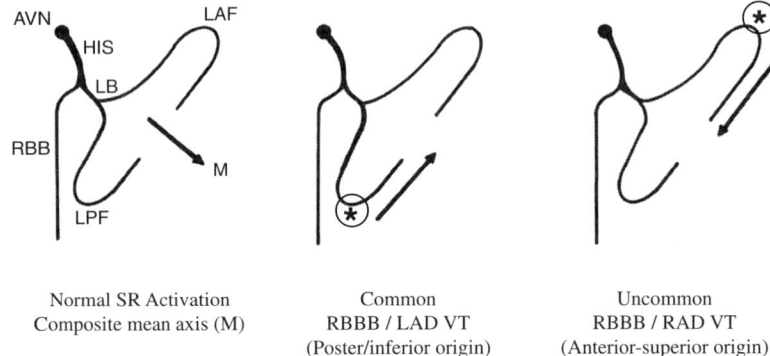

Normal SR Activation	Common	Uncommon
Composite mean axis (M)	RBBB / LAD VT	RBBB / RAD VT
	(Poster/inferior origin)	(Anterior-superior origin)

Figure 13. Idiopathic left ventricular tachycardia. AVN = atrioventricular node; HIS = His bundle; LAF = left anterior fascicle; LAD = left axis deviation; LPF = left posterior fascicle; RAD = right axis deviation; RBBB = right bundle branch block; SR = sinus rhythm; VT = ventricular tachycardia.

strongly supports the suggestion that, in at least some patients, the mechanism of this arrhythmia is microreentry.[86,87] In this particular report, a single radiofrequency energy delivery at the site described abolished tachycardia. The zone of slow conduction in idiopathic left ventricular tachycardia shows tachycardia-dependent conduction delay involving calcium channel-dependent and partly depressed sodium channel conductions.[85]

In some patients, however, burst atrial or ventricular sequences rather than critically timed extrastimuli are required for arrhythmia induction.[88,89] In these patients there is often a history of exercise-related episodes and isoprenaline greatly facilitates induction at electrophysiology testing. The termination of tachycardia in these patients by vagal maneuvers has led to suggestions that distally displaced slow-response nodelike fibers may constitute the anatomical substrate.[90]

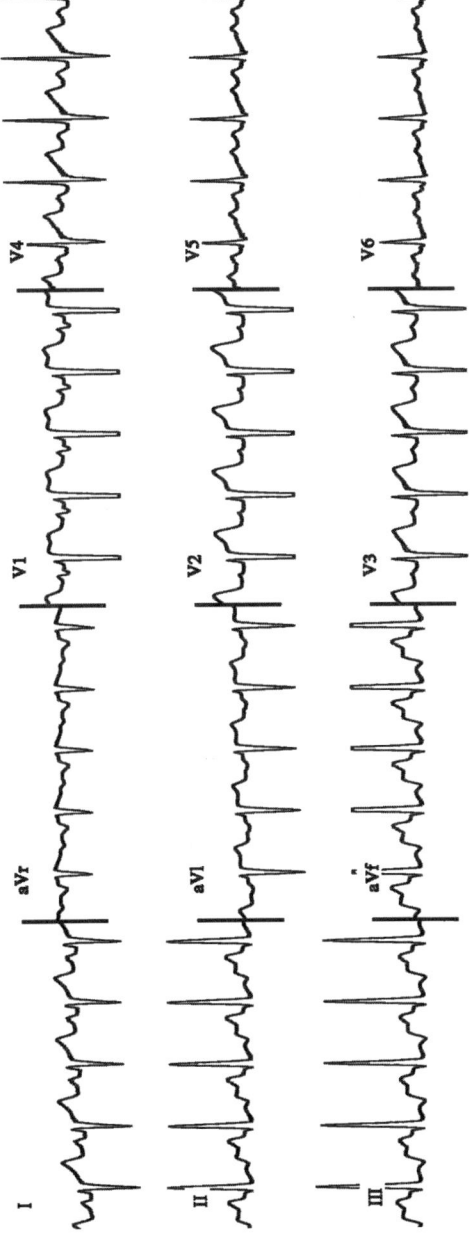

Figure 14. Sinus rhythm ECG in a patient with idiopathic left ventricular tachycardia. Repolarization changes inferiorly (II/III/aVf) shortly after restoration of sinus rhythm in a patient with idiopathic left ventricular tachycardia.

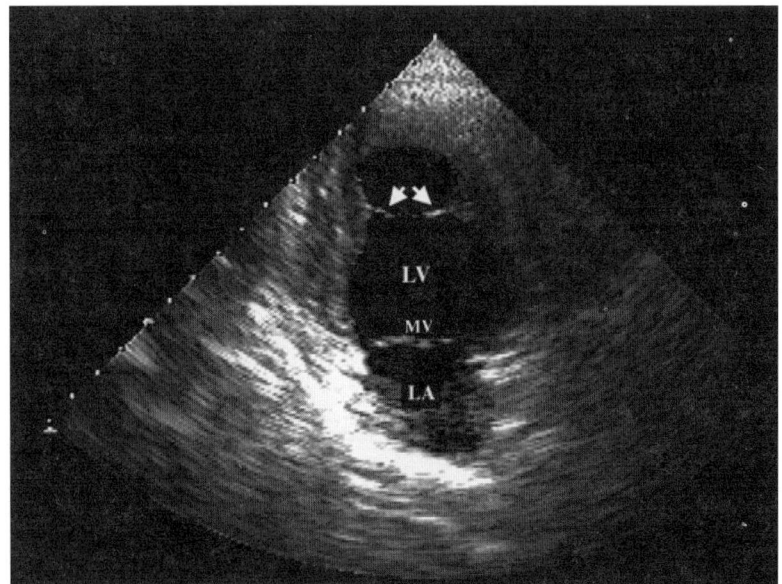

Figure 15. False left ventricular tendon and idiopathic left ventricular tachycardia. Apical four-chamber echocardiogram showing a false tendon (arrow) apically in the left ventricle with its septal and lateral insertions. MV = mitral valve; LA = left atrium.

The mechanism of idiopathic left ventricular tachycardia is therefore debated, with some patients having features more compatible with a triggered automatic or enhanced automatic mechanism and others having features more typical of classic reentry.[48,54,82,91-94] It now seems probable that patients with this form of tachycardia have a spectrum of arrhythmogenic mechanisms accounting for these differences in spontaneous arrhythmia behavior and electrophysiology.[83,86,87]

Another controversial issue is the role of false tendons in the genesis of idiopathic left ventricular tachycardia (Figure 15).[95-100] The evidence is contradictory at present. From a series of 15 patients with this form of ventricular tachycardia, and 671 control subjects undergoing echocardiography, Thakur et al[95] concluded that a false tendon was a consistent finding in patients with this arrhythmia, but only present in 5% of controls. These authors hypothesized that the false tendon could either provide an anatomical pathway for reentry or facilitate nonreentrant arrhythmias by stretching the Purkinje fiber network. In contrast, Lin et al[96] concluded that a left ventricular fibromuscular band was not a specific substrate for this arrhythmia, since although they found one in 17 of 18 patients with the arrhythmia, they also found one in 35 of 40 control subjects undergoing investigation for paroxysmal supraventricular tachycardia.

Purkinje Potentials and Catheter Ablation of Idiopathic Left Ventricular Tachycardia

The common right bundle branch, left axis deviation form of this arrhythmia originates near the left posterior fascicle in the inferolateral or midseptal region of the left ventricle. The site is sufficiently consistently one quarter to one third the distance from apex to base to begin mapping the arrhythmia at this site (Figure 16). In this region a specialized Purkinje spike potential is usually recorded and precedes QRS activation both in sinus rhythm and during tachycardia, indicating the location of the conducting fascicle (Figure 17). In sinus rhythm the specialized signal precedes QRS onset by 5 to 10 ms. If catheter stability and reliable capture can be obtained, pacing at these sites provides an identical 12-lead QRS match of the clinical tachycardia.

30° RAO projection   40° LAO projection

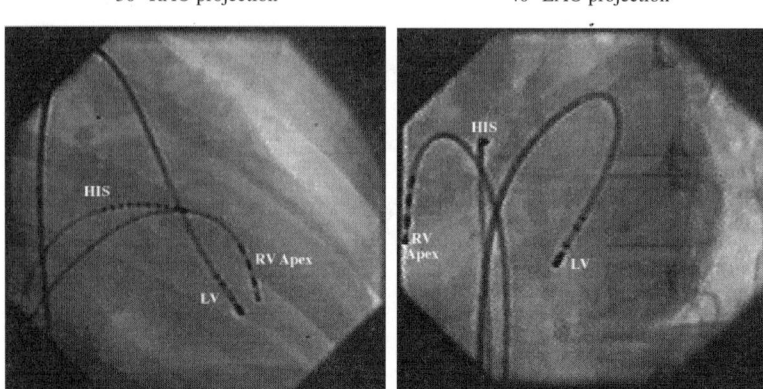

Figure 16. Idiopathic left ventricular (fascicular) tachycardia. Bi-plane x-rays showing the site of successful ablation of idiopathic left ventricular tachycardia (LV). A decapolar catheter is in the His position (HIS) and a quadpolar catheter at the right ventricular apex (RV Apex).

Catheter ablation is now the treatment of choice in patients with symptoms, and these specialized potentials can be used to guide the procedure (Figure 18).[10,101-104] In patients with a false tendon in the left ventricle, the successful ablation site has been shown to be close to its septal insertion.[95] When Purkinje potentials are recorded at several sites in the area of interest, ablation should be directed to the site of earliest recording.[55,102-104] However, in some reports the site of ultimate tachycardia ablation was where the specialized and local myocardial electrogram fused. Success rates of 85% to 93% for catheter ablation of idiopathic left ventricular tachycardia have been reported from relatively small series.[10] Following successful ablation, some patients show hemi-block on their ECG in sinus rhythm compatible with destruction of all conductions over the left posterior fascicle.[105]

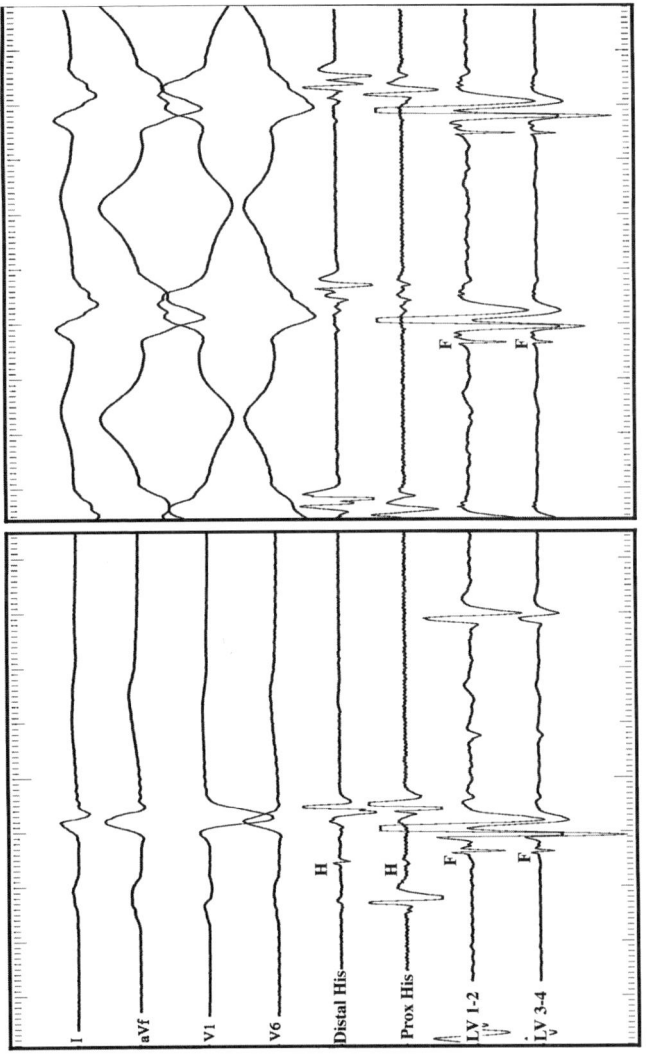

Figure 17. Idiopathic left ventricular (fascicular) tachycardia. Panels show four surface ECG channels, two His recording channels, and proximal and distal bipolar recordings from the ablation catheter in sinus rhythm (left) and in tachycardia (right). A prominent specialized potention (F) is recorded in both. It precedes each QRS in tachycardia and follows His activation in sinus rhythm, with identical F-V timing in both.

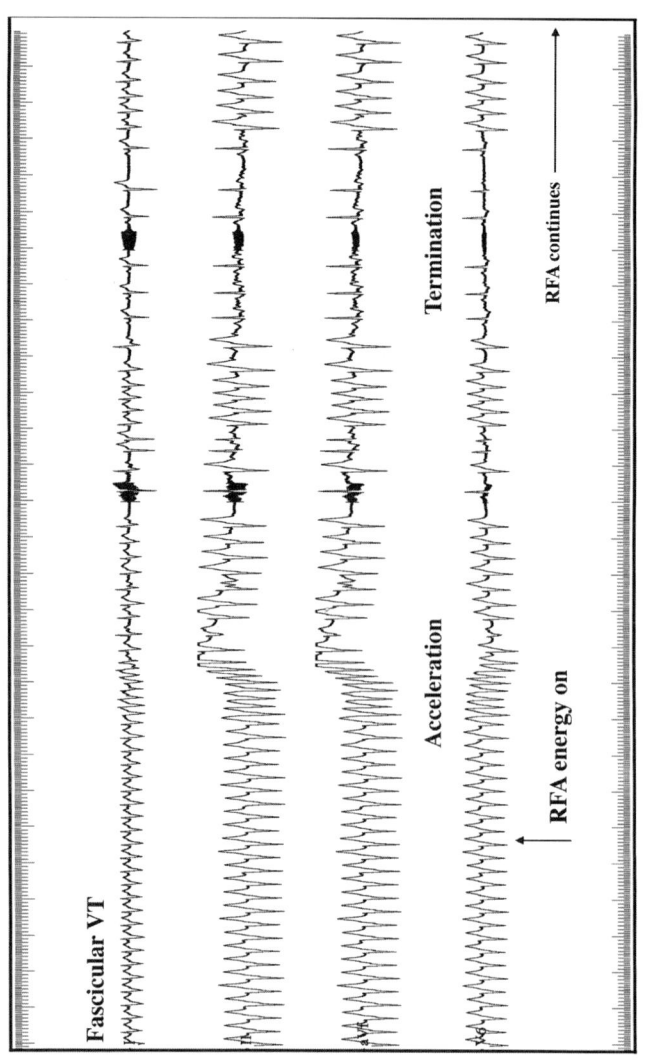

Figure 18. Idiopathic left ventricular (fascicular) tachycardia. Successful ablation in a patient with idiopathic left ventricular tachycardia. With the onset of energy delivery, tachycardia accelerates to termination. Intermittent runs of irregular, slower tachycardia were observed until energy delivery ceased. VT = ventricular tachycardia; RFA = radiofrequency ablation.

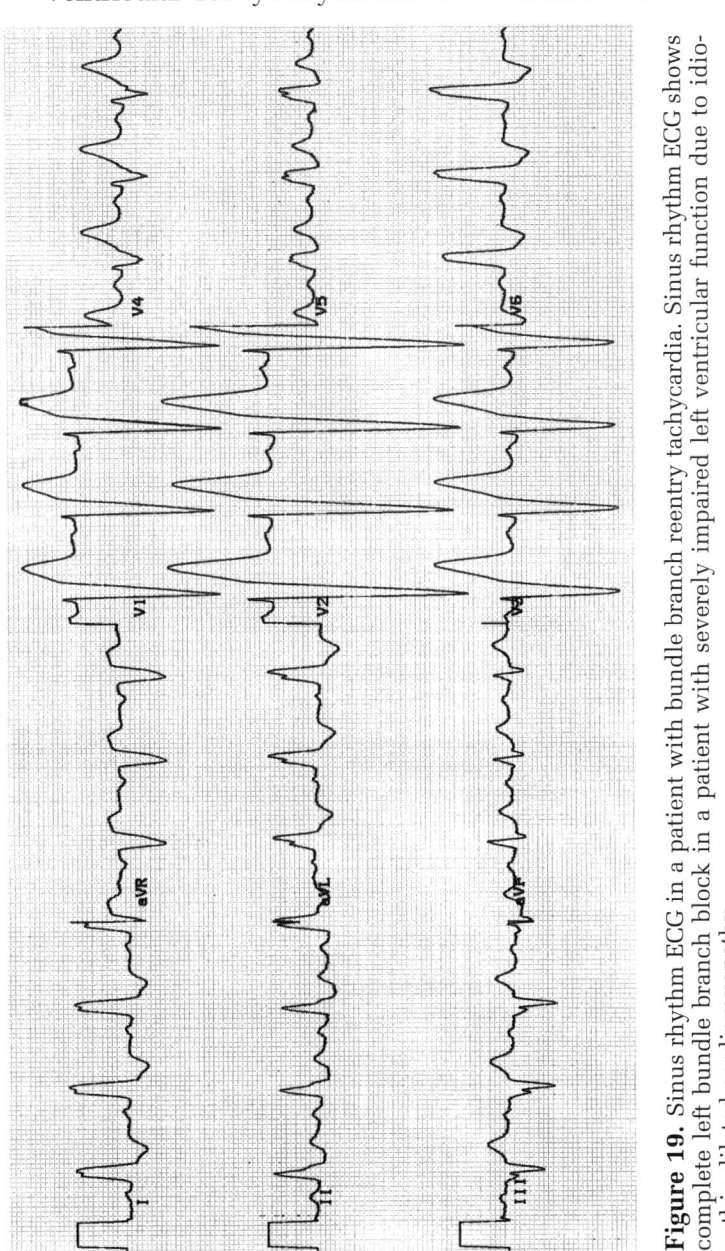

Figure 19. Sinus rhythm ECG in a patient with bundle branch reentry tachycardia. Sinus rhythm ECG shows complete left bundle branch block in a patient with severely impaired left ventricular function due to idiopathic dilated cardiomyopathy.

Bundle Branch Reentrant Ventricular Tachycardia

Sustained bundle branch reentrant ventricular tachycardia is a highly malignant arrhythmia predominantly reported in patients with advanced left ventricular dysfunction. Prognosis for patients with this form of ventricular tachycardia is poor, due primarily to the severity of coexisting left ventricular failure. In one series of 42 patients followed for a mean of only 15.8 months, the mortality rate was 55%. The causes of death in the 23 patients were: congestive cardiac failure, 31%; sudden, presumed arrhythmic death, 10%; nonsudden cardiac death, 7%; and noncardiac death, 7%.[106] Bundle branch reentry tachycardia has been reported rarely in the context of a structurally normal heart[106] but as a mechanism for sustained ventricular tachycardia due to primary conduction tissue disease, it merits discussion. In advanced cardiac disease, nonsustained forms of bundle branch reentry are said to be common but sustained forms accounted for only 6% of ventricular tachycardia ablation in one series.[107] Even then, they usually coexist with other forms of ventricular tachycardia unrelated to the bundle branch reentrant mechanism.[108] Although in typical patients with sustained bundle branch reentry tachycardia, the prognosis is determined as much by the degree of left ventricular dysfunction as by the arrhythmias themselves, arrhythmias alone would likely determine prognosis in a patient with a normal heart.

The cause of left ventricular dysfunction in a typical patient with bundle branch reentrant ventricular tachycardia is usually either advanced coronary artery disease or idiopathic dilated cardiomyopathy. There is usually a history of clinical heart failure and the ECG typically shows conduction abnormalities such as left bundle branch block, first-degree heart block, or nonspecific interventricular conduction delay (Figure 19). Sustained forms of this arrhythmia have also been described in patients with Ebstein's anomaly and hypertrophic obstructive cardiomyopathy. Although small numbers of patients with no identifiable cardiac disease are included in each series, their natural history and outcome are not separated out from the remainder.[106,107,109]

The arrhythmia usually presents with a hemodynamic comprising ventricular tachycardia and syncope or with cardiac arrest. The 12-lead ECG of sustained tachycardia almost always has a left bundle branch morphology, although a right bundle branch block variant is rarely described.[106]

Electrophysiology of Bundle Branch Reentry Ventricular Tachycardia

The tachycardia circuit includes the His bundle, the right and left bundle branches, the Purkinje system, and the ventricular myocardium. Figure 20 shows the typical circuit and illustrates how differences in refractory periods of the bundles are exploited by spontaneous ectopy to cause sustained ventricular tachycardia. Isolated cases of interfascicular reentry have also been described either in isolation or coexisting with other forms of specialized conduction tissue reentry (Figure 21).[105,106,109]

At electrophysiology study in these patients, there is always evidence of advanced conduction tissue disease with the HV interval in sinus rhythm typically exceeding 80 ms.[110] Short-long pacing sequences typically induce tachycardia, and induction may be facilitated by isopren-

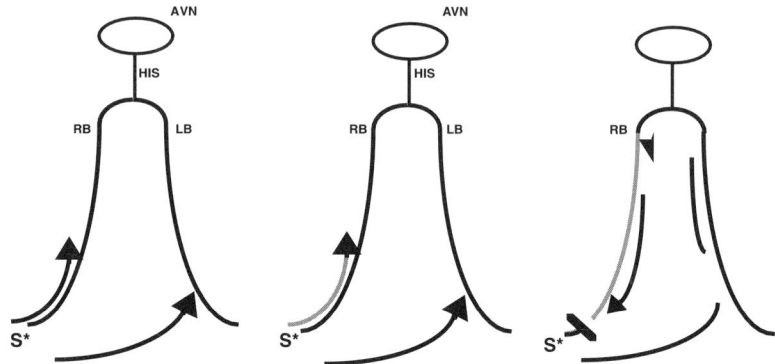

Figure 20. The reentry circuit in bundle branch reentry tachycardia. The circuit in typical bundle branch reentry tachycardia includes the His bundle, right (RB) and left (LB) bundle branches, as well as ventricular myocardium. Differences in refractory periods of the diseased bundles are exploited by spontaneous ectopy to initiate and maintain tachycardia. AVN = atrioventricular node.

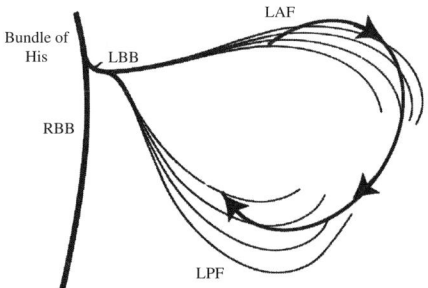

Figure 21. Interfascicular reentry tachycardia. Reentry occurring between left anterior and left posterior fascicles of the left bundle. The right bundle branch is a bystander to this circuit, but may be implicated in other tachycardias in the same patient.

aline or class I antiarrhythmic agents. Tachycardia can usually be terminated by rapid ventricular pacing.

If the arrhythmia is suspected, multiple catheters should be sited to record proximal and distal His, right,

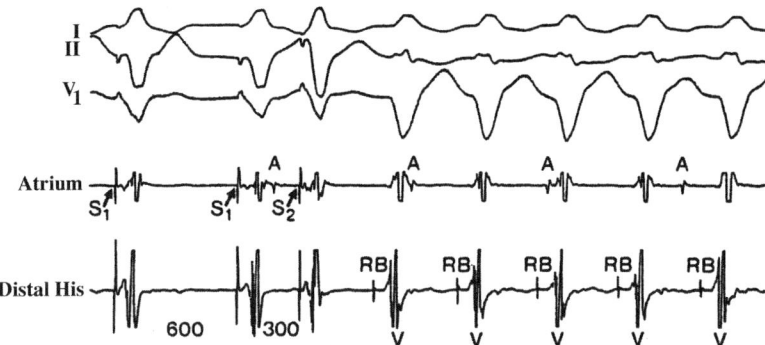

Figure 22. Typical bundle branch reentry tachycardia. Induction of left bundle branch block morphology ventricular tachycardia by programmed ventricular stimulation (S_1/S_2). There is a ventriculoatrial dissociation and each QRS is preceded by a right bundle potential (RB), confirming that this is the antegrade limb of the circuit.

and left bundle potentials. During the typical left bundle branch form of tachycardia, specialized conduction potentials from the His bundle and right bundle branch precede ventricular activation. The retrograde limb is over the left bundle (Figure 22). Any irregularity in the HH interval precedes any irregularity in the VV interval. The uncommon right bundle branch block morphology of bundle branch reentry tachycardia in which the circuit is reversed is also illustrated (Figure 23).

Findings Suggestive of Bundle Branch Reentry Tachycardia

The following findings should heighten suspicion of bundle branch reentry tachycardia and prompt the siting of catheters to record the activation sequence of the specialized conduction system in tachycardia:

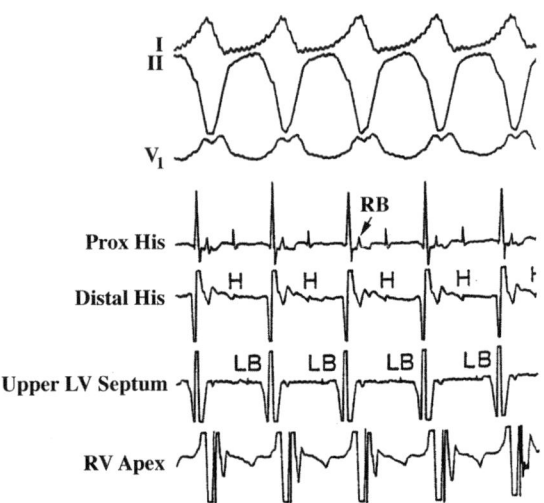

Figure 23. Uncommon form of bundle branch reentry tachycardia. Right bundle branch morphology of tachycardia. Each QRS is preceded by a His and left bundle branch (LB) potential, and followed by a right bundle branch (RB) potential, confirming the direction of the circuit's activation.

1. Any patient with idiopathic dilated cardiomyopathy and poorly tolerated ventricular tachycardia.
2. Any patient with ventricular tachycardia whose HV interval in sinus rhythm is prolonged.
3. Any inducible monomorphic ventricular tachycardia with left bundle branch block QRS morphology.
4. Any ventricular tachycardia in which QRS activation is preceded by His or other specialized potentials.

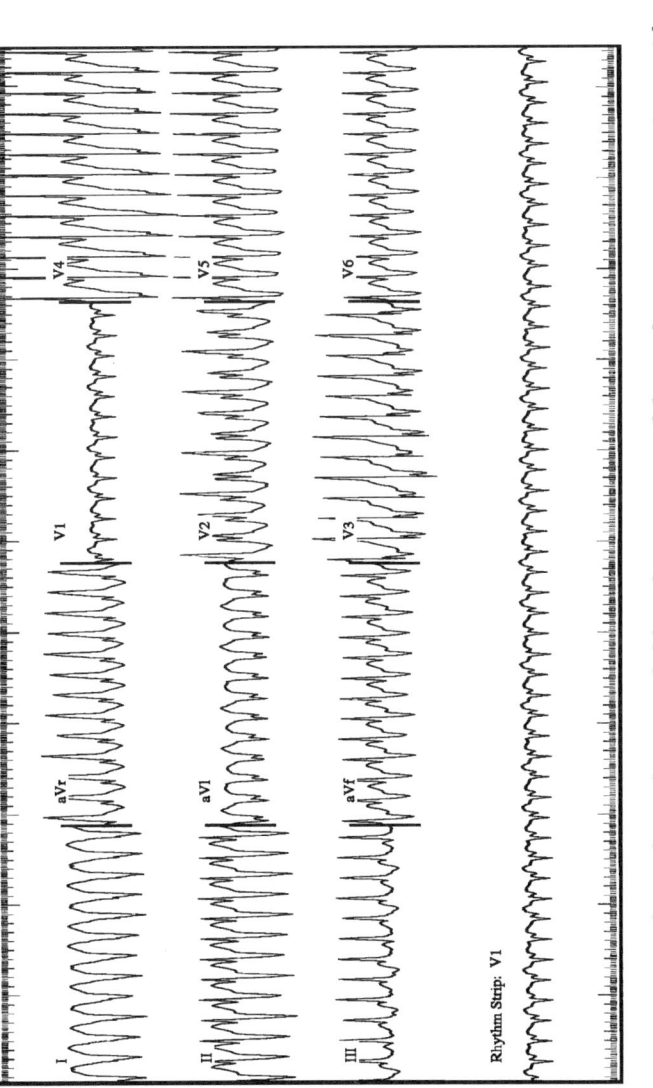

Figure 24. Ventricular tachycardia in a child without structural heart disease. In comparison with the adult patient, ventricular tachycardia is more likely to have 1:1 VA association, a shorter cycle length, and a disconcertingly narrow QRS. Adenosine administration led to transient VA dissociation in this example (note leads III/V_1).

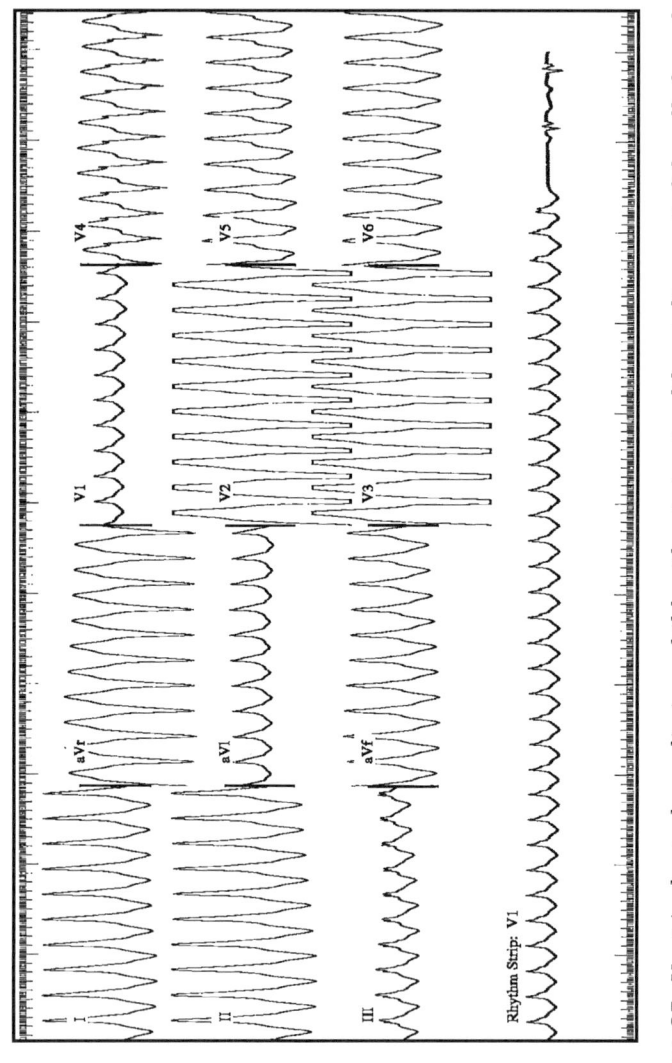

Figure 25. Ventricular tachycardia in a child without structural heart disease. Left bundle branch block ventricular tachycardia with 1:1 ventriculoatrial association. Restoration of sinus rhythm by a single spontaneous ventricular ectopic beat (rhythm strip) suggests a reentrant mechanism.

Catheter Ablation in Bundle Branch Reentrant Tachycardia

In bundle branch reentry tachycardia, both right and left bundles are essential components of the circuit. Ablation of the right bundle therefore abolishes tachycardia by creating a site of absolute block in the circuit. The recommended site for right bundle branch block ablation is distal to the point where the maximum amplitude of the His deflection is recorded, in order to avoid causing a deterioration in AV conduction.[111]

As previously mentioned, however, these patients commonly have other ventricular tachycardias coexisting with their bundle branch reentry and right bundle ablation should not be seen as anything other than a palliative treatment aimed at reducing the frequency of arrhythmia episodes. The finding of bundle branch reentry therefore requires careful examination for the presence of other arrhythmia mechanisms which may pose an equal life threat. Even after right bundle ablation, defibrillator implantation is often needed to provide overall control of the different forms of ventricular arrhythmias induced in these patients.[110] Sometimes it is preferable to ablate the left bundle branch when this is the more diseased of the two main bundles, in order to avoid causing a deterioration in AV conduction that requires permanent pacing.[109,112] Berger et al[109] reported a patient who, after ablation of the right bundle, was still capable of sustained tachycardia due to interfascicular reentry. This was abolished after ablation of the left posterior fascicle of the left bundle (Figure 21).

Pediatric Ventricular Tachycardias

Ventricular tachycardias can occur in the fetus and in children of all ages.[113-116] There is, however, considerable reluctance to make this diagnosis in pediatric patients, especially if there is no history of congenital heart disease. Yet, the single most common category of children with ventricular tachycardia have "normal hearts."[117-119] Difficulties in diagnosis are compounded by an absence of symptoms in the high proportion of children with this arrhythmia, which usually has a relatively narrow QRS configuration and 1:1 ventriculoatrial conduction (Figure 24).[120] In children, neither the rate of tachycardia nor the presence or absence of symptoms are of any value in distinguishing supraventricular from ventricular tachycardia. However, the arrhythmia's response to intravenous bolus adenosine may be particularly helpful, especially if it produces ventriculoatrial dissociation without tachycardia termination (Figure 25).

There are so many potential causes of ventricular tachycardia in children that a classification just on the basis of the arrhythmia is of limited clinical value in defining prognosis or guiding management. As in the adult age group, however, children suspected of having ventricular tachycardia should have organic cardiac disease excluded at an early stage, and the context in which the arrhythmia occurs provides some framework for management.[120] The main heart conditions to be excluded in children with ventricular tachycardia include: (1) congenital heart disease (eg, tetralogy of Fallot, Ebstein's anomaly, coronary anomalies, and mitral valve prolapse); (2) hypertrophic or dilated cardiomyopathy including arrhythmogenic right ventricular dysplasia; (3) acquired arrhythmias due to factors such as cardiac tumors, post-surgical connections, or those precipitated by drug therapies; and (4) those due to abnormalities of cardiac repolarization such as the congenital long QT syndrome and variants.

In contrast, the occurrence of ventricular fibrillation in a child previously considered healthy is more likely to lead to an appropriate referral for specialist attention. The management of such patients is best guided by issues raised in the later sections of this volume on the congenital long QT syndrome and idiopathic ventricular fibrillation.[113,118,121]

Investigations in the Pediatric Patients with Ventricular Tachycardia

In addition to obtaining ECG documentation of the abnormal arrhythmia and its response to interventions (eg, bolus adenosine therapy), a 12-lead ECG in sinus rhythm, transthoracic echocardiogram, chest x-ray, and exercise test complete the noninvasive assessment. Most children with symptoms due to sustained ventricular tachycardia have an underlying cardiac abnormality and this helps classify them in a clinically useful way. For example, ventricular tachycardia occurring after correction of tetralogy of Fallot characterizes a child as having a reentrant form of ventricular tachycardia related to postoperative scar. The circuit is usually located in the interventricular septum or right ventricular outflow region. The prognosis can be related to series of such patients in the literature and management can be guided by the arrhythmia's response to short-term drug testing.

Catheter or surgical ablation or defibrillator therapy are also appropriate for some patients in this group.[122] As previously mentioned, unlike adults, the single most common group of children with ventricular tachycardia are those with normal hearts.[114] However, the group defined in this way is rather heterogeneous and includes children with specifically pediatric forms as well as with all of the tachycardia mechanisms seen in adults. The most common reason for specialist referral is the identification of a fast heart rate in an asymptomatic child. Clearly, the presence or absence of symptoms depends to some extent on the child's ability to provide an independent history. Some children, however, experience symptoms of palpitation, dizziness, and frank syncope. Up to half of all pediatric patients with ventricular tachycardia can have their arrhythmias reproduced by an exercise stress test.[119] Induction by exercise is a marker of risk, even in the absence of structural heart disease, but serial tests can be used to evaluate drug treatments.[123]

Invasive electrophysiology testing is of particular value in children without exercise-precipitated arrhythmias who have sufficient symptoms to justify therapy. Defining the arrhythmia as precisely as possible in terms of its electrophysiology profile and mechanism as well as its site of origin may provide additional guidance for treatment. In addition, the opportunity provided by invasive electrophysiology to abolish the arrhythmia by catheter ablation is another reason to undertake it in selected cases.

Incessant Ventricular Tachycardia in Infancy and Early Childhood

When ventricular tachycardia is present for more than 10% of a 24-hour period, it is defined as incessant. Incessant ventricular tachycardia is rare but presents dramatically with either progressive cardiac failure, cardiovascular collapse, or even cardiac arrest. This type of arrhythmia is frequently present for more than 80% of the time, and in the past was considered refractory to drug treatment. Neither the rate nor ECG morphology is diagnostic but ventriculoatrial dissociation is often present or can be unmasked by adenosine administration, thus clarifying its ventricular origin.

In the past, because of its refractoriness to drug therapy and its hemodynamic impact, some affected children underwent surgical ablation of the origin. In one series of 21 surgically treated patients, a myocardial abnormality was visible at the site of origin of tachycardia in 12.[124,125] Biopsy of the site of origin showed hemangiomas (Purkinje cell tumors) in 13 and rhabdomyomas in two. There are now also reports of successful catheter ablation of these arrhythmias in infants.[126]

In recent years, however, amiodarone and flecainide have been effective in controlling these incessant ventricular tachycardias, obviating the need for ablative therapy.[127,128] When required, even the use of flecainide and amiodarone in combination appears safe in this pediatric population.[129]

Despite its worrisome initial presentation, one of the most intriguing aspects of this arrhythmia is its apparent spontaneous resolution over time. This also argues for a conservative strategy of management based on drug therapy in all but the most refractory cases. Several series now report the success of discontinuation of drug therapy after periods of about 2 years without reemergence of tachycardia.[129,130]

It is important to distinguish the aforementioned hemodynamically compromised group from asymptomatic children who have slower forms of ventricular arrhythmias of short duration in the absence of structural heart disease. These children usually come to attention coincidentally. The rate of their tachycardia can vary from accelerated junctional rhythm-type behavior with normal QRS morphology just exceeding the sinus cycle length to broader QRS tachycardias at faster rates. There is little evidence that these arrhythmias require treatment and in the absence of structural heart disease they are considered innocent and self-limiting.

Cyclic AMP-Mediated and Idiopathic Left Ventricular Tachycardia in Children

Cyclic AMP-mediated right ventricular outflow tract and idiopathic left ventricular (fascicular) tachycardias are now also described in patients in the pediatric age group.[117,131-133] While these tachycardias are equally amenable to catheter ablation, the potential for complications from the procedure and their benign prognosis suggest that curative procedures be delayed until the child is of reasonable size and weight, except in exceptional circumstances.[134-137]

Normal heart ventricular tachycardia in pediatric patients is increasingly recognized and is due to diverse etiologies, including some of the types also seen in adults.[132,133,138] The prognosis is largely determined by the etiology whether related to trivial structural heart disease, the congenital long QT syndrome, or having a truly idiopathic basis. Management must be individualized to the arrhythmia and ranges widely from, at one extreme, no requirement for therapy, through the need for aggressive drug treatment for a short period, to a requirement for curative catheter ablation of a persisting problem, to drug and/or defibrillator therapy for the more malignant forms of the long QT syndrome. For a more detailed review of the topic beyond the scope of this volume, refer to Wren (1996).[120]

Catecholaminergic Polymorphic Ventricular Tachycardia in Children ("Bidirectional Ventricular Tachycardia")

Life-threatening ventricular tachyarrhythmias are rare in childhood in the absence of structural heart disease. Several primarily electrical abnormalities have been identified to explain some of these arrhythmias, including the congenital long QT syndromes, Brugada syndrome with right bundle branch block and persistent ST segment elevation (see below), and a short coupled variant of torsade de pointes.[139,140] Bidirectional ventricular tachycardia is another highly malignant but even rarer syndrome, which, although initially described in the 1970s, has only recently been characterized.[141,142]

Children with this arrhythmia typically present with recurrent syncope triggered by exercise or emotion in the 3- to 16-year age range. They are often mistakenly thought to have epilepsy, and as a result, the cardiac diagnosis is delayed. No genetic studies are available on patients to date, but one third have a family history of either recurrent syncope or sudden death.[143,144] The relationship, if any, of this syndrome to the congenital long QT syndrome remains to be determined. The importance of identifying this rare condition is that both the arrhythmia and the associated symptoms can be abolished by β-blockade. Nadolol is considered the preferred agent because of its long half-life and greater potency. Without β-blockade, mortality is estimated to be 50% before age 20.[142] Amiodarone is less effective in sudden death prevention, and class I antiarrhythmic drugs are contraindicated.

These children do not have structural heart disease, their QT interval is normal (QTc ≤ 400 ms), but they have a resting sinus bradycardia (typically 60 to 70 beats/min). The diagnosis is made on Holter ECG recordings during exercise or from recordings during an incremental infusion of isoprenaline, where a typical pattern is described.[142] Sinus rate initially increases to approximately 120 to 130 beats/min, but is then overtaken by a narrow QRS accelerated junctional arrhythmia. As stress increases, monomorphic ventricular ectopy beings and becomes increasingly complex. At higher levels of stress, bursts of monomorphic, bidirectional, and polymorphic ventricular tachycardia occur, which ultimately progress to longer and longer runs of a ventricular fibrillation-like rhythm, with hemodynamic collapse and syncope. After cessation of stress, the pattern reverses over the same time course as it began (Figure 26). The efficacy of therapy can be assessed by its ability to prevent the sinus rate from reaching the threshold of 120 to 130 beats/min, required for arrhythmia induction, at peak exercise or isoprenaline stress (Figure 27).

Acquired bidirectional ventricular tachycardia has been described in the context of digitalis intoxication[145,146] and, rarely, in other forms of poisoning,[147]

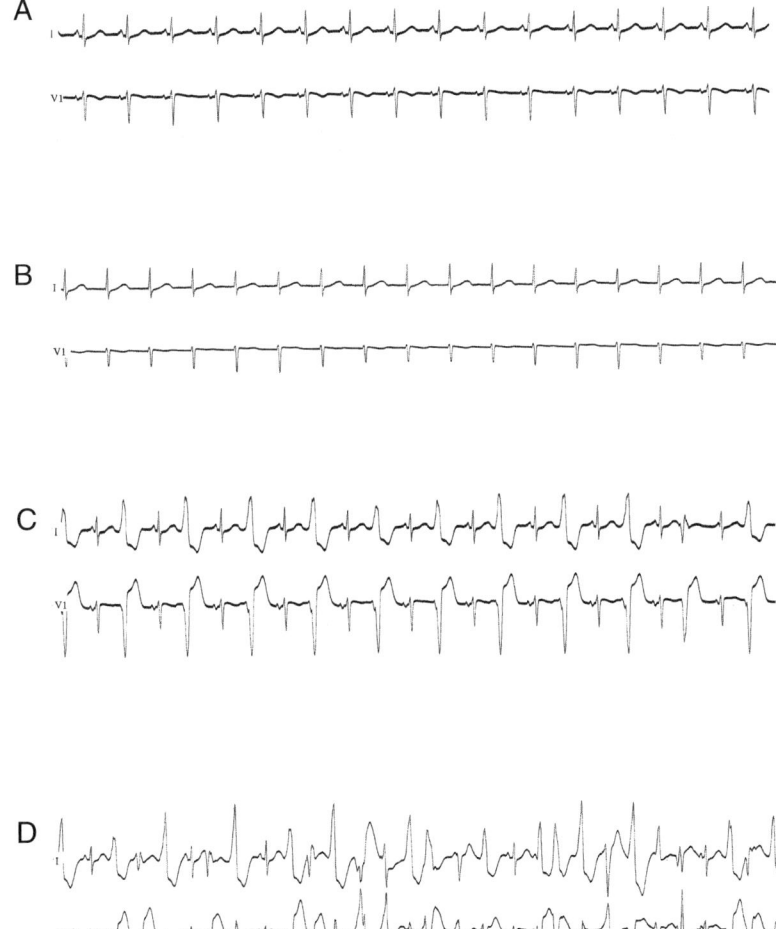

Figure 26. Bidirectional tachycardia. Response to incremental isoprenaline infusion. **A.** Sinus tachycardia. **B.** Accelerated junctional
rhythm. **C.** Monomorphic ventricular ectopy. **D.** Polymorphic bidirectional ventricular tachycardia. I am indebted to Dr. C. Wren, Freeman
Hospital, for this illustration.

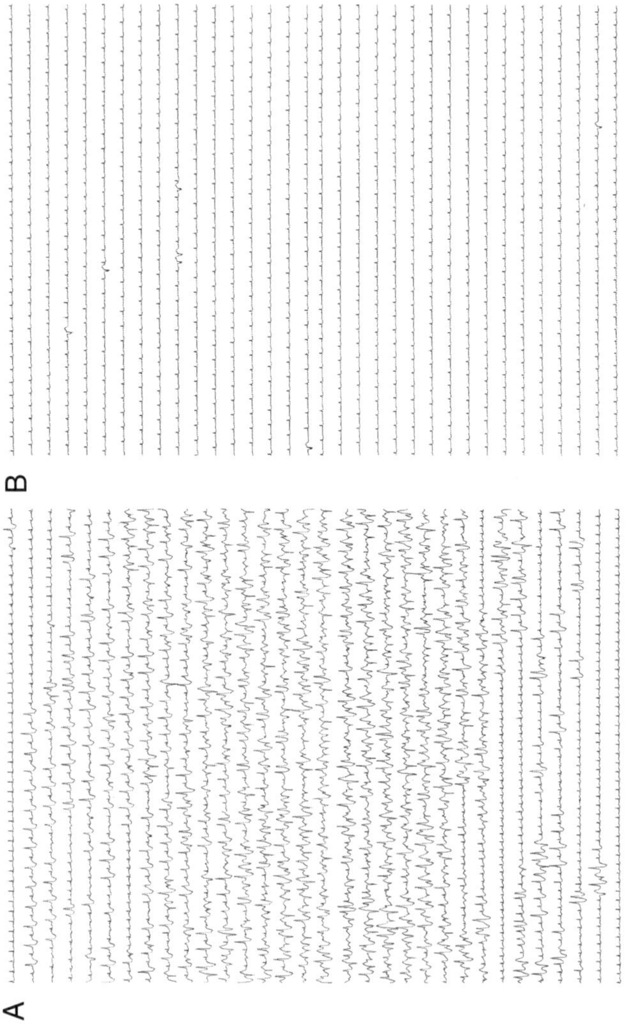

Figure 27. Bidirectional ventricular tachycardia. Response to incremental isoprenaline infusion without (A) and with (B) β-blockade. I am indebted to Dr. C. Wren, Freeman Hospital, for this illustration.

where the treatment is supportive until the offending agent can be eliminated.

Idiopathic Ventricular Fibrillation

Ventricular fibrillation usually occurs in severely diseased hearts either as a degeneration from more organized ventricular tachycardia or de novo when the heart's own antifibrillatory mechanisms are reduced or have been overwhelmed.[148] The prognosis in patients who survive the first episode is partly determined by the risk of arrhythmia recurrences and partly by the severity of the underlying structural heart disease—left or right ventricular dysfunction, coronary artery disease, or left ventricular hypertrophy. The relative contributions of arrhythmic and cardiac causes to subsequent mortality vary. For example, correcting a large ischemic burden by coronary bypass grafting in a patient without prior infarction would be expected to reduce both the risk of arrhythmia recurrences and infarction without involving any specifically "antiarrhythmic" measures. In contrast, bypass grafting alone is unlikely to be sufficient to prevent further arrhythmias in patients with extensive left ventricular scar due to prior myocardial infarction. In this instance, antiarrhythmic measures such as defibrillator implantation with or without antiarrhythmic drug therapy or antiarrhythmic surgery are required. When arrhythmia recurrences are not preventable and pose a life threat, the implantable cardioverter defibrillator is highly effective in preventing sudden death independent of the underlying etiology.[149] The basic principle of management, therefore, is that where the cause of spontaneous ventricular fibrillation is understood, efforts should be

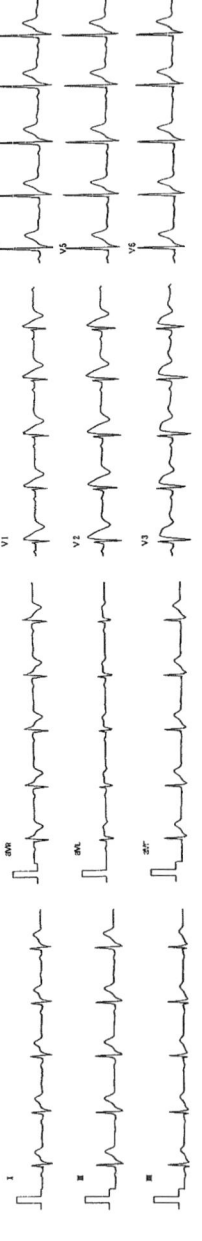

Figure 28. Sinus rhythm ECG of a patient with idiopathic ventricular fibrillation. Note the abnormal pattern of ST segment elevation in the right precordial leads (V_1 through V_3) and repolarization abnormality. This pattern identifies one subgroup of "normal heart" patients at particularly high risk of ventricular fibrillation (Brugada syndrome). The ECG features can sometimes be unmasked when not present by intravenous procainamide or ajmaline.

directed primarily at correcting or reducing the risk of recurrences. Such measures might include initiation of angiotensin-converting enzyme inhibitor therapy or valve replacement to improve left ventricular dysfunction, anti-ischemic and lipid-lowering treatments in patients with ischemic heart disease, correction of electrolyte disturbances, or stopping therapies responsible for drug-induced arrhythmias.

These general principles also apply to the 5% of patients without structural heart disease who are resuscitated from ventricular fibrillation.[13,31,150] Of 194 survivors of out-of-hospital cardiac arrest undergoing electrophysiology evaluation in one study, only 6 (3%) had idiopathic ventricular fibrillation.[151] The condition is therefore rare but, unlike in other subgroups, prognosis is likely to be determined almost exclusively by arrhythmia recurrences.[152]

Since idiopathic ventricular fibrillation is a diagnosis of exclusion, it can only be reached after extensive evaluation to detect other causes.[153,154] It may be impossible at times to decide whether cardiac abnormalities detected after prolonged resuscitation were the cause of or caused by the arrhythmic event. Changes such as diffuse repolarization abnormalities, anterior left ventricular hypokinesis, left bundle branch block, or hypokalemia after resuscitation may cause confusion, especially when no previous records are available for comparison.

Blood toxicology screen may help to identify arrhythmias that are due to cocaine-induced coronary spasm, for example, or to substance abuse where the history might not be forthcoming.[155-159]

The terms *normal heart* and *idiopathic ventricular fibrillation* are likely to become increasingly imprecise, as minor abnormalities identified only by cine-MRI of the heart are increasingly identified in these patients.[160] At most hospitals with specialist arrhythmia management services, survivors of idiopathic ventricular fibrillation are treated with implantable cardioverter defibrillators[161] and information on the prognosis is based almost exclusively on small retrospective series of patients treated in this way.[152,162] The incidence of arrhythmia recurrences is controversial but in one study of 28 patients followed for a mean of 30 months, 57% experienced shock therapy from their devices,[163] and in another series of 19 patients, 37% experienced major recurrences during follow-up of 41 months.[152] Shock frequency in this type of patient, however, is lower than that in patients with devices for arrhythmias of other etiologies.[149,164,165] Others have suggested a role for antiarrhythmic drug therapy alone in some of these patients using class IA agents,[166] β-blockers,[167,168] or calcium channel blockers.[169,170] A means of using electrophysiology testing to evaluate therapy responses in these patients has even been suggested,[154,168] although not universally accepted.[14] However, because these patients are usually younger than those with arrhythmias due to left ventricular dysfunction, the lifestyle and cost implications of long-term device therapy is considerable.

Recognizable Subsets of Patients with Idiopathic Ventricular Fibrillation

Brugada Syndrome

A subset of survivors of ventricular fibrillation with "structurally normal hearts" are those with the pattern of ST segment elevation in the right precordial leads on their sinus rhythm ECG.[4,171-173] The ECG abnormality and its association with recurrent cardiac arrests or sudden death has been labeled *Brugada syndrome* (Figure 28).[174] More than 60 patients with these features have now been reported in the world literature and the high recurrence in those who survive the initial episode makes the implantable cardioverter defibrillator the treatment of choice at the present time. Intermittent forms of the syndrome have also been described with transient normalizations of the ECG. The typical abnormalities can, however, be unmasked in these patients by the administration of class lA antiarrhythmic agents such as procainamide.[4] It is of particular concern that some patients with typical ECG features have been described who only developed arrhythmias subsequently. It now therefore seems advisable to treat any asymptomatic patients as if they had already experienced arrhythmias and to screen first-degree relatives of all clinical cases.[4]

The likely importance of Brugada syndrome is further emphasized by the recent finding that 59% of 27 male Thai survivors studied with the sudden unexplained death syndrome had the ECG features of the condition.[175] On the basis of the results of pharmacological interventions, it has been hypothesized that the ECG features might be due to an area that has repolarized early or remained "depolarized" in the right ventricle.[174,176]

How Idiopathic is Idiopathic Ventricular Fibrillation?

As increasing numbers of patients with ventricular fibrillation and structurally normal hearts are being identified and treated with defibrillator therapy, some clinical subgroups seem to be emerging. These include: (1) the

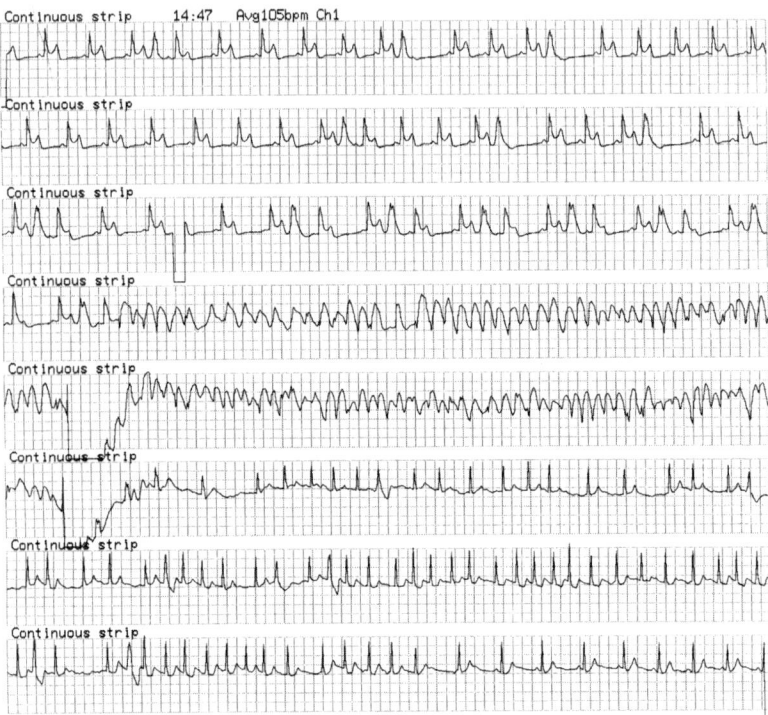

Figure 29. Idiopathic ventricular fibrillation in a patient with normal coronary arteries. Note the progressive ST segment elevation, QRS widening, and increasingly frequent ventricular ectopy prior to ventricular fibrillation. An implanted cardioverter defibrillator fails to restore sinus rhythm with its first shock but succeeds with the second.

identification of Brugada syndrome as a subgroup at potential risk of sudden death; (2) the documentation of ST segment elevation in the absence of obstructive coronary disease prior to ventricular fibrillation in others (Figure 29)[177,178]; (3) the recognition that some patients without a long QT interval behave as if they had[140,179,180]; (4) the detection of minor right ventricular abnormalities on cine-MRI imaging[69,160] in some; and (5) increased echogenicity in the basal interventricular septum on echocardiography in others.

The identification of such subgroups is likely to lead ultimately to the development of specific therapies and, possibly, to less reliance on defibrillator therapy. However, much remains unknown at present. For example, whether focal right ventricular abnormalities progress to a more extensive cardiomyopathy or remain localized and amenable to electrical inactivation remains to be determined.

The Long QT Syndrome: Congenital and Acquired Forms

Congenital Long QT Syndrome

In recent years, significant advances in our understanding of the underlying abnormalities responsible for the inherited long QT syndromes have emerged.[181-183] The mechanism of torsade de pointes and ventricular fibrillation in the congenital long QT syndrome is explained by early and possibly late afterdepolarizations and triggered activity due to repolarization abnormalities.[184-187] From recent evidence, the primary abnormality appears to be at a cell membrane receptor level, and a growing number of genetically distinct types are being identified, some of which even have different ECG patterns of QT prolongation.[188] The genetic abnormalities identified to date still account for only a minority of patients with sporadic forms of the syndrome. However, they do provide clues as to why some patients do not respond to conventional β-adrenergic blockade.[23,189-191] The traditional emphasis on autonomic cardiac sympathetic imbalance as the underlying cause of the syndrome and the arrhythmias associated with it is no longer adequate, although sympathetic surges appear to play a particular arrhythmia-triggering role in some patients.[192] Presently, therefore, β-adrenergic blockade, preferably with nadolol, remains the recommended first-line treatment. There is still controversy over the next appropriate treatment for patients who do not respond to this, and over the best first therapy for those in whom β-blockade is absolutely contraindicated. Increasingly, implantable defibrillator therapy is advised in preference to the older recommendation of surgical or chemical cardiac denervation procedures. The recent genetic information suggests a possible future role for nicorandil and mexiletine in certain specific genetically identifiable subgroups. Although it is premature to use these agents in place of β-blockade, observation of QT responses to trials of different pharmacological agents may provide a way to characterize long QT syndrome patients at the time of initial diagnosis.

Despite recent advances, however, the congenital long QT syndrome remains a highly malignant condition if untreated, with a mortality of 60% to 70% over 10 to 15 years of follow-up from the first syncope.[193] Appropriate therapy with β-adrenergic blockade reduces the 15-year sudden death rate to 3% to 5%.[194,195]

While typical forms of the long QT syndrome are readily identifiable from the 12-lead surface ECG both by their prolonged rate corrected QT interval and widened QT dispersion, there are also categories of patients who manifest the same torsade de pointes-like ventricular arrhythmias but whose QT interval is "normal." Some of these patients can have abnormalities of QT behavior unmasked by longer term recordings or by stress evaluations. Failure of appropriate QT shortening on exercise or intermittent increases in the QT interval prior to arrhythmias are evident in some.[196-198] The relationship of these normal-QT patients to those with typical long QT syndrome probably depends on understanding the fundamental cell membrane receptor abnormalities for the two populations.[199,200] For a comprehensive up-to-date discussion of this syndrome the reader is referred to other works by Schwartz.[1a,192]

Acquired Long QT Syndrome

Myocardial repolarization is affected by a very large number of factors including autonomic cardiac innervation, electrolyte concentrations—particularly intracellular calcium and potassium—and a bewildering array of drug treatments including those for cardiac and noncardiac conditions.[24] The QT interval on ECG is also prolonged in medical conditions such as Parkinson's disease,[201] liver impairment,[202] anorexia nervosa,[203] and starvation, and in patients on liquid protein diets.[204] Whether drug-induced QT prolongation[203] results in clinical arrhythmias may therefore depend on the coming together of variables such as individual susceptibility for genetic or gender reason, drug-induced bradycardia, coexisting medical conditions, and the triggering factors of electrolyte disturbances on bradycardia.[202-206]

The occurrence of torsade de pointes and other proarrhythmic reactions to drugs that prolong repolarization is appreciably higher in women than in men in all studies of gender differences, and suggests that females are more susceptible.[207] Many of the reports of arrhythmogenic reactions attributable to antiarrhythmic drug therapies are, of course, in patients with advanced structural heart disease, impaired left ventricular function, and coronary artery disease. The precipitation of life-threatening ventricular tachyarrhythmias as a result of the use of antiarrhythmic drugs for benign atrial arrhythmias such as paroxysmal atrial fibrillation and other forms of intra-atrial reentry or for asymptomatic nonsustained ventricular tachycardia is of particular concern.[208] Particular care should therefore be exercised in antiarrhythmic prescribing for this type of patient.

QT prolongation without an increase in QT dispersion about the heart is probably antiarrhythmic. Increased QT dispersion (QT_{max} minus QT_{min}) is the hallmark of drug-induced proarrhythmia due to altered repolarizations (Figure 30).[209]

The mechanism of arrhythmias in the acquired long QT syndrome is attributed to occurrence of early afterdepolarizations and early afterdepolarization-induced triggered activity.[210] For arrhythmias to occur, three ingredients are required: (1) critical prolongation of repolarization; (2) a net depolarizing current carrying the charge for the early afterdepolarization; and (3) propagation of the early afterdepolarizations to the rest of the heart. At a cellular level, drug-induced arrhythmias mediated through early afterdepolarizations act predominantly by one of three mechanisms. They cause a delay in one or both potassium currents IK and IK1, an increase in the transsarcolemmal calcium current (ICa), or a delay of sodium current (INa) inactivation. The typical arrhythmia observed is torsade de pointes, with its classic short-long-short induction sequence (Figures 31 and 32). Whenever this arrhythmia is observed, drug-induced proarrhythmia should be suspected and all medications reviewed.

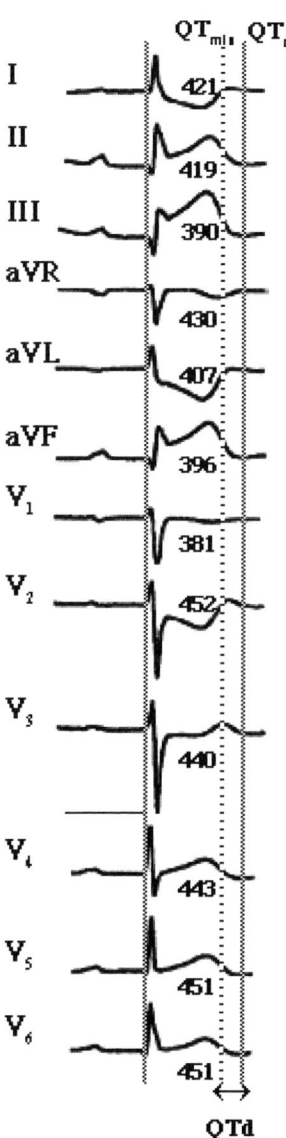

Figure 30. QT interval dispersion about the standard 12-lead ECG. QTd = QT_{max} minus QT_{min}. QT dispersion is a better measure of proarrhythmic potential than QT maximum.

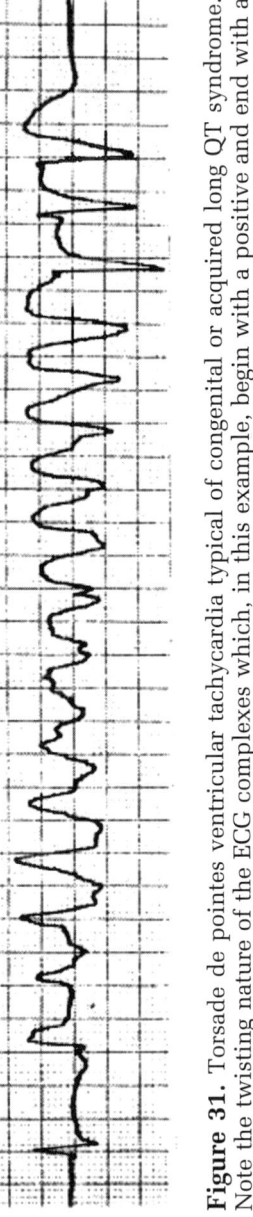

Figure 31. Torsade de pointes ventricular tachycardia typical of congenital or acquired long QT syndrome. Note the twisting nature of the ECG complexes which, in this example, begin with a positive and end with a negative QRS axis.

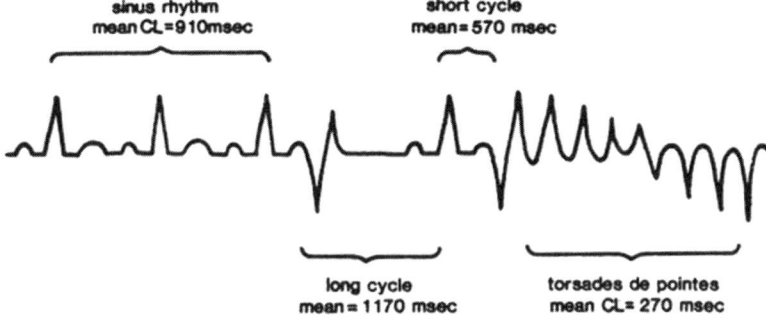

sinus rhythm
mean CL=910msec

short cycle
mean=570 msec

long cycle
mean = 1170 msec

torsades de pointes
mean CL= 270 msec

Figure 32. Initiation of torsade de pointes ventricular tachycardia. Note the "short-long-short" coupling intervals prior to tachycardia initiation.

Proarrhythmic Effects of Antiarrhythmic Agents

The proarrhythmic effects of antiarrhythmic drugs are now well recognized and can occur either as idiosyncratic reactions or in situations of drug toxicity in patients with or without cardiac disease (Figure 33).[211-214] Class I antiarrhythmic agents have long been associated with arrhythmogenic reactions. Class Ic agents (flecainide, encainide, propafenone)[215,216] are more likely to cause proarrhythmia than class Ia agents (quinidine, procainamide, disopyramide) which, in turn, are more likely to cause this problem than class Ib drugs (lignocaine, mexiletine). Patients with depressed left ventricular function and previously documented life-threatening arrhythmias are most susceptible.[217] Typical torsade de pointes-type arrhythmogenic reactions are seen both with class Ia and class III agents and facilitated by hypokalemia and bradycardia. Essentially, torsade de pointes can be produced by all antiarrhythmic agents that prolong myocardial repolarization and increase its

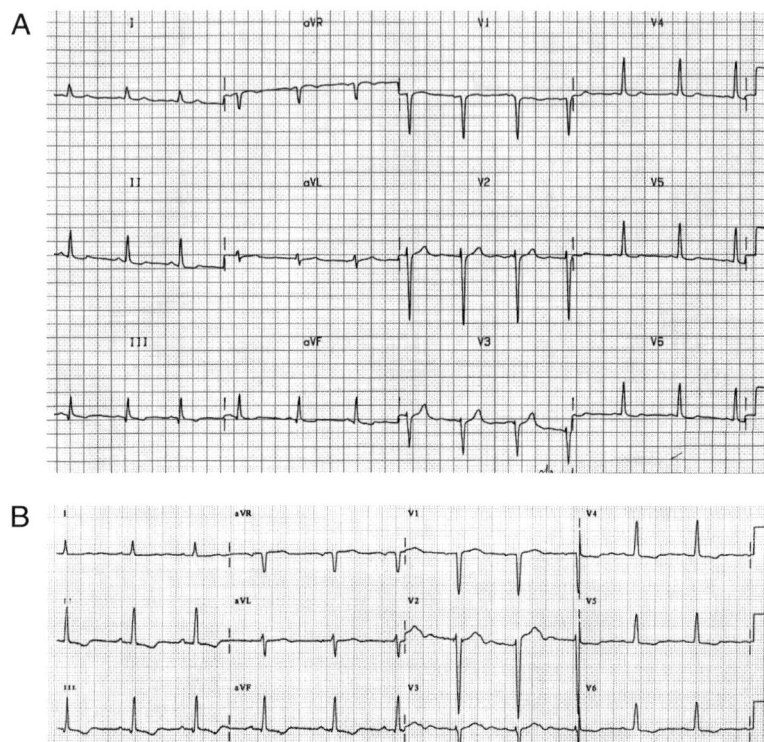

Figure 33. QT prolongation by drug therapy (**A**) before amiodarone and (**B**) after amiodarone loading. This pair of ECGs shows QT prolongation and increased QT dispersion with amiodarone therapy in a patient with cardiomyopathy. These changes preceded an increase in spontaneous arrhythmias requiring drug withdrawal.

dispersion about the heart, although the precise incidence varies with different agents.

Class I Antiarrhythmic Agents

Most reports of confirmed arrhythmogenesis relate to quinidine, disopyramide, and procainamide.[218] Where quinidine is regularly used, it is one of the most common causes of the acquired long QT syndrome and an incidence of arrhythmogenic reaction of 1.5% per year is quoted.[219] Several reports have highlighted a number of features common to patients experiencing proarrhythmia with this agent. In one study[219] it was noted that quinidine proarrhythmia tended to occur in patients prescribed the agent for nonsustained ventricular tachycardia, atrial fibrillation, or atrial flutter. In those treated for atrial fibrillation, the torsade-like rhythm tended to occur after conversion to sinus rhythm. Although most reports of arrhythmia occurred within days of starting the agent, some patients alarmingly experienced torsade de pointes after long-term therapy, possibly due to the development of hypokalemia.

Sotalol, d-Sotalol, and Amiodarone

Reports of torsade de pointes with sotalol,[220,221] d-sotalol,[222] and amiodarone[223-226] and dofetilide[227] are less common than with class I agents. In one report which summarized the results of 65 English-language case reports of torsade de pointes related to amiodarone treatment, a 2% overall incidence of proarrhythmic effects and a 0.7% incidence of torsade de pointes was documented.[224] The authors concluded that this very low incidence of proarrhythmic effects combined with the negligible inotropic effect of the drug made it particularly suited to the prevention of sudden death.[228]

Nonantiarrhythmic Cardiovascular Therapies

The role of cardiovascular drug therapy in facilitating or causing sudden death in a variety of contexts remains unknown. In one population-based study of patients treated for essential hypertension in the absence of other heart diseases, those who experienced a primary cardiac arrest were reviewed and compared to controls, who were also hypertensive. Resting ECGs were reviewed in order to estimate the severity of left ventricular hypertrophy, extent of any myocardial injury, and degree of QT prolongation. In comparison of the 80th with the 20th percentile score for QT interval duration, the risk of cardiac arrest was increased 80%, with odds ratios of 1.8 and 95% confidence intervals 1.3 to 2.7.[229]

Some antianginal agents may affect myocardial repolarization. For example, the potassium channel opener, nicorandil, shortens repolarization and could therefore facilitate arrhythmias, particularly in ischemic myocardium in humans as in animal preparations.[230] However, there have been no reports of proarrhythmia attributable to nicorandil in humans to date despite extensive use of the drug.[231,232] Even β-adrenergic blockers, such as metoprolol, in standard therapeutic doses[233] have been associated with the development of delayed ventricular repolarization. The issue of the etiology of QT prolongation is further complicated in patients with coronary artery disease since there have even been rare reports of QT prolongation and torsade de pointes arrhythmias as the sole manifestation of ischemia.[234]

Drug-Induced QT Prolongation and Torsade de Points in Noncardiac Drug Treatments

A bewildering and seemingly ever-increasing list of drugs used for all manners of noncardiac indications are now known to effect myocardial repolarizations and cause QT prolongation. Cases of torsade de pointes-like arrhythmias and ventricular fibrillation have been reported for many of them, confirming the clinical relevance of the problem. Spectacular examples of arrhythmogenicity of QT prolongation are provided by the drugs lidoflazine,[235] prenalamine,[236] and terodiline.[237] These examples of an antiarrhythmic, an antianginal, and a bladder-stabilizing agent, respectively, were all mediated through QT prolongation. The seriousness and frequency of the arrhythmogenic reactions led to each agent being withdrawn because of the occurrence of ventricular tachyarrhythmias de novo. Even sudden death in alcoholic patients without evidence of structural heart disease is attributable to QT prolongation.[238] The antimicrobials spiromycin,[239] used in toxoplasmosis prophylaxis, and ampicillin,[240,241] under circumstances of anaphylaxis, have also caused QT prolongation with ventricular proarrhythmia. A full review of the diverse drug reports is beyond the scope of this volume; however, Table 3 gives some examples to highlight the extent of present concerns and the different families of drugs implicated to date. It is not intended as a comprehensive list. The following examples highlight some of the difficulties in evaluating or anticipating adverse drug reactions with serious cardiac consequences and underscore some of the mechanisms involved.

Erythromycin

Intravenous erythromycin causes QT prolongation and has been associated with torsade de pointes-like reactions. In one study in which microelectrode and whole cell, patch clamp techniques were used to assess the dif-

Table 3

Classification and Some Examples of Acquired Long QT Syndrome

Medical conditions	anorexia nervosa/starvation/liquid protein diets
	Parkinsons disease
	liver disease
	intracranial bleeding/craniotomy
	cardiomyopathies
	ischemia (rare sole manifestation)

Drug-Induced

Cardiovascular therapies

Antiarrhythmics

class Ic > Ia > Ib	flecainide; encainide;
	propafenone; quinidine;
class III	procainamide; disopyramide;
	sotalol; d-sotalol; amiodarone;
	dofetilide

Antianginal/antihypertensives/lipid-lowering agents
β-blockers (metoprolol)
potassium channel openers
(nicorandil)
ketanserin
probucol

Noncardiovascular therapies

Antibiotics/Antimicrobials	erythromycin; spiramycin
	ampicillin (anaphylaxis)
	ketoconazole
Psychoactive Agents	major tranquilizers
	(phenothiazines)
	antipsychotics (sertindole)
	seditives/antiphychotic
	(haloperidol)

Table 3

Continued

	SSRIs antidepressants (doxepin; peroxetine) tricyclic antidepressants (desiprimine/imiprimine)
Antiemetic Agents	5-HT$_3$ serotonine antagonists (ondansetron; topisetron)
Antireflux Agents	cisapride[244]
Antihistamines	terfenadine; astemizole
Miscellaneous Other	organophosphate[245]/arsenic[246] poisoning

SSRIs = serotonin uptake inhibitors

ferent effects of erythromycin on epicardial, endocardial, and M-cells in transmural strips, arterially perfused wedge preparations and single myocytes, a preferential response of M-cells to class III reactions of erythromycin, were identified.[242] This was due principally to the effect of the drug on inhibiting IK(r) in a population of cells without IK(s) receptors. This preferential effect of prolonging M-cell repolarization resulted in a prominent dispersion of repolarization across the ventricular wall. Polymorphic ventricular tachycardia was readily and reproducibly inducible once erythromycin was added compared to the same preparation without the drug.

In another study of 44 critically ill patients, the acute effects of intravenous erythromycin on the QT interval of 44 critically ill patients was studied. In contrast to control traces, the QT interval was significantly prolonged on ECG recordings after infusion, although no patient experienced arrhythmias.[243] However, when the complexity of drug regimens in critically ill patients is considered, the possibilities for synergistic effects to prolong myocardial repolarizations and increase its heterogeneity is substantial. Consider, for example, the arrhythmogenic potential of the standard drug regimen in an immune, compromised patient receiving combination chemotherapy or HIV treatments. Antibiotic, antifungal, antiviral, and antiemetic elements are not uncommon, not to mention the impaired nutritional status, electrolyte abnormalities, and multiorgan compromise often coexisting in these patients.[206] Even if ventricular arrhythmias occurred in this context, the likelihood is that they would be attributed to the patients' overall status rather than to a specific drug. If, however, the observed arrhythmia was torsade de pointes, drug-facilitated arrhythmia should be considered and the therapy regimen reviewed.

Psychoactive Drugs

Tricyclic antidepressants are well known for their arrhythmogenic potential. Although no significant arrhythmias were observed in one retrospective study of 36 adult patients taking desipramine or imipramine in a variety of drug doses or in a small study in pediatric patients, others have shown marked increases in absolute and rate-corrected QT intervals with low-dose tricyclic treatment in adults.[244,245] A possible link between QT prolongation and reports of sudden death in these patients has been suggested.[245] Torsade de pointes is a hazard of long-term treatment with ketanserine.[246] In a study comparing two newer antidepressants, fluoxetine and doxepin, in patients with major depressive orders, doxepin but not fluoxitine was noted to significantly prolong the corrected QT interval. The authors suggested that fluoxetine, therefore, had a greater safety margin when antidepressants were required in patients with concomitant cardiac diseases.[247]

Haloperidol, a drug frequently used to control acutely agitated or delirious patients in medical and surgical wards, has a reputation for cardiac safety. However, it too can cause torsade de pointes-like reactions in sensitized patients by prolonging repolarization.[205] Phenothiazines have also been implicated in arrhythmias.[248]

In summary, many drugs prescribed for both cardiac and noncardiac indications prolong myocardial repolarization. The risk of developing life-threatening ventricular arrhythmias as a result is real and the literature abounds in case reports relating to specific agents. Women are more likely to experience the problem than men and aggravating factors include hypokalemia, bradycardia, and comorbidity. The fact that drugs used for reflux esophagitis,[249] infection,[239,240,242,243] bladder stabilization,[237] emesis,[250] and a wide range of psychiatric indications[205,244,246-248] can result in arrhythmias is of concern, but should not paralyze prescribing. The occurrence of torsade de pointes in any patient should immediately lead to the suspicion of a drug-induced arrhythmia and an urgent review of all therapy. The mainstays of treatment include withdrawal of the agent implicated, correction of bradycardia by temporary pacing if necessary, and correction of hypokalemia where appropriate.

Conclusion

Ventricular tachycardia can and does occur in patients without evidence of structural heart disease. Our knowledge of many of these arrhythmias is incomplete and the distinctions based on their fundamental mechanisms will undoubtedly become clearer within the next 5 years. Cyclic AMP-mediated, idiopathic left ventricular, and bundle branch reentry tachycardias are under intense study at present because they can be cured at low risk by radiofrequency catheter ablation. Because of their unusual electrical behavior, cyclic AMP-mediated and idiopathic left ventricular tachycardias are shedding new light on our understanding of the mechanisms of ventricular tachyarrhythmias in humans. The distinction between these arrhythmias, which usually have a benign prognosis, occurring in the context of a normal heart contrasts with the poor prognosis of patients with other forms of ventricular tachyarrhythmias. Exclusion of organic heart disease is an essential part of the evaluation of these patients and methods for approaching this have been suggested.

Despite occurring as primary electrical disease in structurally normal hearts, idiopathic ventricular fibrillation and congenital and acquired long QT syndromes stand out as potentially lethal conditions calling for more aggressive management. The framework for thinking about these arrhythmias suggested by this volume will undoubtedly change and date quickly. However, it is hoped that the reader will find this synopsis useful as an introduction to the topic and that it will prove a useful starting point from which to build on future reports and advances in our knowledge as they unfold.

References

1a. Schwartz PJ. The Long QT Syndrome. A. John Camm (ed). Armonk, NY: Futura Publishing Co., 1997.

1b. Bhadha K, Marchlinski FE, Iskandrian AS. Ventricular tachycardia in patients without structural heart disease. Review. Am Heart J 1993;126(5): 1194–1998.

2. Goy JJ, Tauxe F, Fromer M, et al. Ten-years followup of 20 patients with idiopathic ventricular tachycardia. PACE 1990;13(9):1142–1147.

3. Sebastien P, Waynberger M, Beaufils P, et al. Isolated ventricular tachycardia without patent cardiopathy. in French. Arch Mal Coeur Vaiss 1976; 69(9):919–928.

4. Brugada J, Brugada P. What to do in patients with no structural heart disease and sudden arrhythmic death? Am J Cardiol 1996;78(5A):69–75.

5. Garcia LC, Fabregas N, Nalda MA. Idiopathic hypocalcemia and ventricular fibrillation: report of a case. in Spanish. Revista Espanola de Anestesiologia y Reanimacion 1990;37(4):231–233.

6. Fauchier JP, Fauchier L, Babuty D, et al. Idiopathic monomorphic ventricular tachycardia. Review. in French. Arch Mal Coeur Vaiss 1996;89(7):897–906.

7. Brooks R, Burgess JH. Idiopathic ventricular tachycardia. A review. Medicine 1988;67(5):271–294.

8. Schols W, Brachmann J, Schmitt C, et al. Continuous ventricular tachyarrhythmia in patients without detectable organic heart disease: Clinical and electrophysiologic findings. in German. Zeitschrift fur Kardiologie 1989;78(12):790–796.

9. Lokhandwala YY, Smeets JL, Rodriguez LM, et al. Idiopathic ventricular tachycardia—characterisation and radiofrequency ablation. Indian Heart J 1994;46(6):281–285.

10. Wen MS, Yeh SJ, Wang CC, et al. Radiofrequency ablation therapy in idiopathic left ventricular tach-

ycardia with no obvious structural heart disease. Circulation 1994;89(4):1690–1696.

11. Gumbrielle T, Furniss SS, Doig C, et al. Successful ablation of incessant ventricular tachycardia. Eur J Cardiac Pacing Electrophysiol 1994;4:258–261.

12. Zhu DW, Maloney JD, Simmons TW, et al. Radiofrequency catheter ablation for management of symptomatic ventricular ectopic activity. J Am Coll Cardiol 1995;26(4):843–849.

13. Priori SG, Paganini V, Boccalatte L, et al. Idiopathic ventricular fibrillation: From a collection of clinical cases to a prospective evaluation. The U-CARE Steering Committee. Unexplained Cardiac Arrest Registry of Europe. in Italian. Giornale Italiano di Cardiologia 1995;25(2):149–158.

14. Li HG, Thakur RK, Yee R, et al. The value of electrophysiologic testing in patients resuscitated from documented ventricular fibrillation. J Cardiovasc Electrophysiol 1994;5(10):805–809.

15. Molander N. Sudden natural death in later childhood and adolescence. Arch Dis Child 1982;57(8): 572–576.

16. Driscoll DJ, Edwards WD. Sudden unexpected death in children and adolescents. J Am Coll Cardiol 1985;5(6 suppl):118B–121B.

17. Neuspiel DR, Kuller LH. Sudden and unexpected natural death in childhood and adolescence. JAMA 1985;254(10):1321–1325.

18. Niimura I, Maki T. Sudden cardiac death in childhood. Jpn Circ J 1989;53(12):1571–1580.

19. Loire R, Tabib A. Unexpected sudden cardiac death. An evaluation of 1000 autopsies. in French. Arch Mal Coeur Vaiss 1996;89(1):13–18.

20. Bacci M, Giusti G. Diagnostic possibilities and limitations of the necropsy examination on cadavers exhumed because of sudden cardiac death. in Italian. Pathologica 1996;88(1):25–28.

21. Bharati S, Lev M. The conduction system findings in sudden cardiac death. J Cardiovasc Electrophysiol 1994;5(4):356–366.

22. Schwartz PJ, Periti M, Malliani A. The long QT syndrome. Am Heart J 1975;89(3):378–390.

23. Towbin JA, Li H, Taggart RT, et al. Evidence of genetic heterogeneity in Romano-Ward long QT syndrome. Analysis of 23 families. Circulation 1994; 90(6):2635–2644.

24. Zehender M, Hohnloser S, Just H. QT-interval prolonging drugs: Mechanisms and clinical relevance of their arrhythmogenic hazards. Review. Cardiovasc Drug Ther 1991;5(2):515–530.

25. Fontaine G, Fontaliran F, Frank R, et al. Ventricular dysplasia. Nosology and sudden death. Review. in French. Ann Cardiol Angeiol 1988;37(7):347–355.

26. Iesaka Y, Hiroe M, Aonuma K, et al. Usefulness of electrophysiologic study and endomyocardial biopsy in differentiating arrhythmogenic right ventricular dysplasia from idiopathic right ventricular tachycardia. Heart Vessels 1990;5(suppl):65–69.

27. Nava A, Thiene G, Canciani B, et al. Clinical profile of concealed form of arrhythmogenic right ventricular cardiomyopathy presenting with apparently idiopathic ventricular arrhythmias. Int J Cardiol 1992;35(2):195–206.

28. Rabinowitz AJ, Maloney JD. Survivors of sudden cardiac death: A rational approach to evaluation and therapy of patients surviving ventricular fibril-

lation. Review. Cleve Clin J Med 1992;59(2):166–172.

29. Shumway SJ, Johnson EM, Svendsen CA, et al. Surgical management of ventricular tachycardia. Ann Thorac Surg 1997;63:1589–1591.

30. Kelly PA, Cannom DS, Garan H, et al. The automatic cardioverter-defibrillator: Efficacy, complications and survival in patients with malignant ventricular arrhythmias. J Am Coll Cardiol 1988; 11(6):1278–1286.

31. Anonymous. Survivors of out-of-hospital cardiac arrest with apparently normal heart. Need for definition and standardized clinical evaluation. Consensus Statement of the Joint Steering Committees of the Unexplained Cardiac Arrest Registry of Europe and of the Idiopathic Ventricular Fibrillation Registry of the United States. Review. Circulation 1997;95(1):265–272.

32. Fei L, Statters DJ, Gill JS, et al. Alteration of the QT/RR relationship in patients with idiopathic ventricular tachycardia. PACE 1994;17(2):199–206.

33. Gill JS, de Belder M, Ward DE. Right ventricular outflow tract ventricular tachycardia associated with an aneurysmal malformation: Use of transesophageal echocardiography during low-energy, direct-current ablation. Am Heart J 1994;128(3): 620–623.

34. Proclemer A, Ciani R, Feruglio GA. Right ventricular tachycardia with left bundle branch block and inferior axis morphology: Clinical and arrhythmological characteristics in 15 patients. PACE 1989; 12(6):977–989.

35. Carlson MD, White RD, Trohman RG, et al. Right ventricular outflow tract ventricular tachycardia:

Detection of previously unrecognized anatomic abnormalities using cine magnetic resonance imaging. J Am Coll Cardiol 1994;24(3):720–727.

36. Sugrue DD, Holmes DR Jr, Gersh BJ, et al. Cardiac histologic findings in patients with life-threatening ventricular arrhythmias of unknown origin. J Am Coll Cardiol 1984;4(5):952–957.

37. Morgera T, Alberti AE, Silvestri F, et al. Morphological findings in apparently idiopathic ventricular tachycardia. An echocardiographic haemodynamic and histologic study. Eur J Cardiol 1985;6:323–334.

38. Peters S, Davies MJ, McKenna WJ. Diagnostic value of endomyocardial biopsies of the right ventricular septum in arrhythmias originating from the right ventricle. Jpn Heart J 1996;37(2):195–202.

39. Poll DS, Marchlinski FE, Buxton AE, et al. Usefulness of programmed stimulation in idiopathic dilated cardiomyopathy. Am J Cardiol 1986;58:992–997.

40. Wellens HJ, Schuilenburg RM, Durrer D. Electrical stimulation of the heart in patients with ventricular tachycardia. Circulation 1972;46(2):216–226.

41. Sakurai M, Nishiono T, Yoshida I, et al. Mechanisms of chronic recurrent idiopathic ventricular tachycardia. Jpn Circ J 1988;52(3):272–279.

42. Sung RJ, Keung EC, Nguyen NX, et al. Effects of beta-adrenergic blockade on verapamil-responsive and verapamil-irresponsive sustained ventricular tachycardias. J Clin Invest 1988;81(3):688–699.

43. Lerman BB, Stein KM, Markowitz SM. Adenosine-sensitive ventricular tachycardia: A conceptual approach. Review. J Cardiovasc Electrophysiol 1996;7(6):559–569.

44. Wilber DJ, Baerman J, Olshansky B, et al. Adenosine-sensitive ventricular tachycardia: Clinical characteristics and response to catheter ablation. Circulation 1993;87:126–134.
45. Lerman BB, Belardinelli L, West GA, et al. Adenosine-sensitive ventricular tachycardia: Evidence suggesting cAMP-mediated triggered activity. Circulation 1986;74:270–280.
46. Klein LS, Shih H-T, Hackett K, et al. Radiofrequency catheter ablation of ventricular tachycardia in patients without structural heart disease. Circulation 1992;85:1666–1674.
47. Zipes DP, Foster PR, Troup PJ, et al. Atrial induction of ventricular tachycardia: Reentry versus triggered automaticity. Am J Cardiol 1979;44(1):1–8.
48. Sung RJ, Shapiro WA, Shen EN, et al. Effects of verapamil on ventricular tachycardias possibly caused by reentry, automaticity, and triggered activity. J Clin Invest 1983;72(1):350–360.
49. Nakagawa H, Mukai J, Nagata K, et al. Early afterdepolarizations in a patient with idiopathic monomorphic right ventricular tachycardia. PACE 1993; 16(10):2067–2072.
50. Fei L, Statters DJ, Hnatkova K, et al. Change of autonomic influence on the heart immediately before the onset of spontaneous idiopathic ventricular tachycardia. J Am Coll Cardiol 1994;24(6):1515–1522.
51. Koch DM, Rosenfeld LE. Tachycardias of right ventricular origin. Cardiol Clin 1992;10:151–164.
52. Coggins DL, Lee RJ, Sweeney J, et al. Radiofrequency catheter ablation as a cure for idiopathic tachycardia of both left and right ventricular origin. J Am Coll Cardiol 1994;23(6):1333–1341.

53. Ohe T, Aihara N, Kamakura S, et al. Long-term outcome of verapamil-sensitive sustained left ventricular tachycardia in patients without structural heart disease. J Am Coll Cardiol 1995;25(1):54–58.
54. Bhandari AK, Hong RA, Rahimtoola SH. Triggered activity as a mechanism of recurrent ventricular tachycardia. Br Heart J 1988;59(4):501–505.
55. DeLacey WA, Nath S, Haines DE, et al. Adenosine and verapamil-sensitive ventricular tachycardia originating from the left ventricle: Radiofrequency catheter ablation. PACE 1992;15(12):2240–2244.
56. Tada H, Ohe T, Yutani C, et al. Sudden death in a patient with apparent idiopathic ventricular tachycardia. Jpn Circ J 1996;60(2):133–136.
57. Gill JS, Blaszyk K, Ward DE, et al. Verapamil for the suppression of idiopathic ventricular tachycardia of left bundle branch block-like morphology. Am Heart J 1993;126(5):1126–1133.
58. Silka MJ, Kron J. Radiofrequency catheter ablation for idiopathic right ventricular tachycardia: First, last or only therapy—who decides? Editorial. J Am Coll Cardiol 1996;27(4):875–876.
59. Gumbrielle T, Bourke JP, Doig JC, et al. Electrocardiographic features of septal locations of right ventricular outflow tract tachycardia. Am J Cardiol 1997;79:213–216.
60. Jadonath RL, Schwartzman DS, Preminger MW, et al. Utility of the 12-lead electrocardiogram in localizing the origin of right ventricular outflow tract tachycardia. Am Heart J 1995;130(5):1107–1113.
61. Movsowitz C, Schwartzman D, Callans DJ, et al. Idiopathic right ventricular outflow tract tachycardia: Narrowing the anatomic location for successful ablation. Am Heart J 1996;131(5):930–936.

62. Rodriguez LM, Smeets JL, Timmermans C, et al. Predictors for successful ablation of right- and left-sided idiopathic ventricular tachycardia. Am J Cardiol 1997;79(3):309–314.
63. Morady F, Kadish AH, DiCarlo L, et al. Long-term results of catheter ablation of idiopathic right ventricular tachycardia. Circulation 1990;82(6):2093–2099.
64. Vohra J, Shah A, Hua W, et al. Radiofrequency ablation of idiopathic ventricular tachycardia. Aust N Z J Med 1996;26(2):186–194.
65. Chinushi M, Aizawa Y, Takahashi K, et al. Morphological variation of nonreentrant idiopathic ventricular tachycardia originating from the right ventricular outflow tract and effect of radiofrequency lesion. PACE 1997;20(2 Pt 1):325–336.
66. Hindricks G. The Multicentre European Radiofrequency Survey (MERFS) Investigators of the Working Group on Arrhythmias of the European Society of Cardiology. Complications of radiofrequency catheter ablation of arrhythmias. Eur Heart J 1993; 14(12):1644–1653.
67. Anonymous. Complications of radiofrequency ablation: A French experience. Le Groupe de Rythmologie de la Societe Francaise de Cardiologie. Review. in French. Arch Mal Coeur Vaiss 1996; 89(12):1599–1605.
68. Mukai J, Nakagawa H, Nagata K, et al. Long-term results of catheter ablation for idiopathic ventricular tachycardia originated from the right ventricular outflow. Jpn Circ J 1993;57(10):960–968.
69. Globits S, Kreiner G, Frank H, et al. Significance of morphological abnormalities detected by MRI in patients undergoing successful ablation of right

ventricular outflow tract tachycardia. Circulation 1997;96(8):2633–2640.
70. Lerman BB, Stein KM, Markowitz SM. Idiopathic right ventricular outflow tract tachycardia: A clinical approach. Review. PACE 1996;19(12 Pt 1):2120–2137.
71. Lerman BB, Stein K, Engelstein ED, et al. Mechanism of repetitive monomorphic ventricular tachycardia. Circulation 1995;92(3):421–429.
72. Shibuya T, Kimura M, Oda E, et al. Ventricular arrhythmia with postural dependency. J Electrocardiol 1985;18(3):303–308.
73. Pons M, Beck L, Leclercq F, et al. Chronic left main coronary artery occlusion: A complication of radiofrequency ablation of idiopathic left ventricular tachycardia. PACE 1997;20(7):1874–1876.
74. Lerman BB, Stein KM, Engelstein ED, et al. Adenosine-sensitive left ventricular tachycardia. PACE 1995;18:940. Abstract.
75. Bogun F, El-Atassi R, Daoud E, et al. Radiofrequency ablation of idiopathic left anterior fascicular tachycardia. J Cardiovasc Electrophysiol 1995; 6(12):1113–1116.
76. Kasanuki H, Ohnishi S, Tanaka E, et al. Idiopathic sustained ventricular tachycardia responsive to verapamil: Clinical electrocardiographic and electrophysiologic considerations. Jpn Circ J 1986;50(1):109–118.
77. Lin FC, Finley CD, Rahimtoola SH, et al. Idiopathic paroxysmal ventricular tachycardia with a QRS pattern of right bundle branch block and left axis deviation: A unique clinical entity with specific properties. Am J Cardiol 1983;52(1):95–100.

78. Kasanuki H, Ohnishi S, Hosoda S. Differentiation and mechanisms of prevention and termination of verapamil-sensitive sustained ventricular tachycardia. Am J Cardiol 1989;64(20):46J–49J.

79. Andrade FR, Eslami M, Elias J, et al. Diagnostic clues from the surface ECG to identify idiopathic (fascicular) ventricular tachycardia: Correlation with electrophysiologic findings. J Cardiovasc Electrophysiol 1996;7(1):2–8.

80. Gaita F, Giustetto C, Leclercq JF, et al. Idiopathic verapamil-responsive left ventricular tachycardia: Clinical characteristics and long-term follow-up of 33 patients. Review. Eur Heart J 1994;15(9):1252–1260.

81. Singh B, Kaul U, Talwar KK, et al. Reversibility of "tachycardia-induced cardiomyopathy" following the cure of idiopathic left ventricular tachycardia using radiofrequency energy. PACE 1996;19(9):1391–1392.

82. Okumura K, Matsuyama K, Miyagi H, et al. Entrainment of idiopathic ventricular tachycardia of left ventricular origin with evidence for reentry with an area of slow conduction and effect of verapamil. Am J Cardiol 1988;62(10 Pt 1):727–732.

83. Sethi KK, Manoharan S, Mohan JC, et al. Verapamil in idiopathic ventricular tachycardia of right bundle branch block morphology: Observations during electrophysiologic and exercise testing. PACE 1986; 9(1 Pt 1):8–16.

84. Griffith MJ, Garratt CJ, Rowland E, et al. Effects of intravenous adenosine on verapamil-sensitive "idiopathic" ventricular tachycardia. Am J Cardiol 1994;73(11):759–764.

85. Okumura K, Yamabe H, Tsuchiya T, et al. Characteristics of slow conduction zone demonstrated during entrainment of idiopathic ventricular tachycardia of left ventricular origin. Am J Cardiol 1996; 77(5):379–383.

86. Kottkamp H, Chen X, Hindricks G, et al. Radiofrequency catheter ablation of idiopathic left ventricular tachycardia: Further evidence for microreentry as the underlying mechanism. J Cardiovasc Electrophysiol 1994;5(3):268–273.

87. Kottkamp H, Chen X, Hindricks G, et al. Idiopathic left ventricular tachycardia: New insights into electrophysiological characteristics and radiofrequency catheter ablation. PACE 1995;18(6):1285–1297.

88. German LD, Packer DL, Bardy GH, et al. Ventricular tachycardia induced by atrial stimulation in patients without symptomatic cardiac disease. Am J Cardiol 1983;52(10):1202–1207.

89. Ohe T, Shimomura K, Aihara N, et al. Idiopathic sustained left ventricular tachycardia: Clinical and electrophysiologic characteristics. Circulation 1988; 77:560–568.

90. Buja G, Folino A, Martini B, et al. Termination of idiopathic ventricular tachycardia with QRS morphology of right bundle branch block and anterior fascicular hemiblock (fascicular tachycardia) by vagal maneuvers. Presentation of 4 cases. in Italian. Giornale Italiano di Cardiologia 1988;18(7):560–566.

91. Tai YT, D'Onofrio JP, Bourke JP, et al. Left posterior fascicular tachycardia due to localized microreentry. Eur Heart J 1990;11:949–953.

92. Aizawa Y, Naitoh N, Kitazawa H, et al. Frequency of presumed reentry with an excitable gap in sus-

tained ventricular tachycardia unassociated with coronary artery disease. Am J Cardiol 1993;72(12): 916–921.

93. Lerman BB. Response of nonreentrant catecholamine-mediated ventricular tachycardia to endogenous adenosine and acetylcholine. Evidence for myocardial receptor-mediated effects. Circulation 1993;87(2):382–390.

94. Lau CP. Radiofrequency ablation of fascicular tachycardia: Efficacy of pace-mapping and implications on tachycardia origin. Int J Cardiol 1994;46(3):255–265.

95. Thakur RK, Klein GJ, Sivaram CA, et al. Anatomic substrate for idiopathic left ventricular tachycardia. Circulation 1996;93(3):497–501.

96. Lin FC, Wen MS, Wang CC, et al. Left ventricular fibromuscular band is not a specific substrate for idiopathic left ventricular tachycardia. Circulation 1996;93(3):525–528.

97. Suwa M, Hirota Y, Nagao H, et al. Incidence of the coexistence of left ventricular false tendons and premature ventricular contractions in apparently healthy subjects. Circulation 1984;70(5):793–798.

98. Suwa M, Hirota Y, Kaku K, et al. Prevalence of the coexistence of left ventricular false tendons and premature ventricular complexes in apparently healthy subjects: A prospective study in the general population. J Am Coll Cardiol 1988;12(4):910–914.

99. Gallagher JJ, Selle JG, Svenson RH, et al. Surgical treatment of arrhythmias. Am J Cardiol 1988;61: 27A–44A.

100. Suwa M, Yoneda Y, Nagao H, et al. Surgical correction of idiopathic paroxysmal ventricular tachycar-

dia possibly related to left ventricular false tendon. Am J Cardiol 1989;64(18):1217–1220.
101. Washizuka T, Aizawa Y, Chinushi M, et al. Alternation of QRS morphology and effect of radiofrequency ablation in idiopathic ventricular tachycardia. PACE 1995;18(1 Pt 1):18–27.
102. Nakagawa H, Beckman KJ, McClelland JH, et al. Radiofrequency catheter ablation of idiopathic left ventricular tachycardia guided by a Purkinje potential. Circulation 1993;88(6):2607–2617.
103. Zardini M, Thakur RK, Klein GJ, et al. Catheter ablation of idiopathic left ventricular tachycardia. PACE 1995;18(6):1255–1265.
104. Katritsis D, Heald S, Ahsan A, et al. Catheter ablation for successful management of left posterior fascicular tachycardia: An approach guided by recording of fascicular potentials. Heart 1996;75(4): 384–388.
105. Crijns HJ, Smeets JL, Rodriguez LM, et al. Cure of interfascicular reentrant ventricular tachycardia by ablation of the anterior fascicle of the left bundle branch. J Cardiovasc Electrophysiol 1995;6(6):486–492.
106. Blanck Z, Akhtar M. Ventricular tachycardia due to sustained bundle branch reentry: Diagnostic and therapeutic considerations. Clin Cardiol 1993;16(8): 619–622.
107. Gonska BD, Cao K, Schaumann A, et al. Ventricular macro-reentry tachycardia of the bundle branch type—indications for catheter ablation. in German. Zeitschrift fur Kardiologie 1993;82(2):116–122.
108. Kusniec J, Strasberg B, Birnbaum Y, et al. Bundle-branch reentry tachycardia. Clin Cardiol 1993; 16(12):892–894.

109. Berger RD, Orias D, Kasper EK, et al. Catheter ablation of coexistent bundle branch and interfascicular reentrant ventricular tachycardias. J Cardiovasc Electrophysiol 1996;7(4):341–347.

110. Mehdirad AA, Keim S, Rist K, et al. Long-term clinical outcome of right bundle branch radiofrequency catheter ablation for treatment of bundle branch reentrant ventricular tachycardia. PACE 1995;18(12 Pt 1):2135–2143.

111. Gherarducci G, De Ponti R, Salerno-Uriarte JA, et al. Transcatheter radiofrequency bundle branch ablation in bundle branch reentry ventricular tachycardia: Report of a case. in Italian. Cardiologia 1996; 41(4):369–374.

112. Blanck Z, Deshpande S, Jazayeri MR, et al. Catheter ablation of the left bundle branch for the treatment of sustained bundle branch reentrant ventricular tachycardia. J Cardiovasc Electrophysiol 1995;6(1): 40–43.

113. Pederson DH, Zipes DP, Foster PR, et al. Ventricular tachycardia and ventricular fibrillation in a young population. Circulation 1979;60:988–997.

114. Rocchini AP, Chun PO, Dick M. Ventricular tachycardia in children. Am J Cardiol 1981;47(5):1091–1097.

115. Lopes LM, Cha SC, Scanavacca MI, et al. Fetal idiopathic ventricular tachycardia with nonimmune hydrops: Benign course. Ped Cardiol 1996;17(3): 192–193.

116. Pfammatter JP, Paul T, Kallfelz HC. Recurrent ventricular tachycardia in asymptomatic young children with an apparently normal heart. Eur J Ped 1995;154(7):513–517.

117. Vetter VL, Josephson ME, Horowitz LN. Idiopathic recurrent sustained ventricular tachycardia in children and adolescents. Am J Cardiol 1981;47(2):315–322.

118. Fulton DR, Chung KJ, Tabakin BS, et al. Ventricular tachycardia in children without heart disease. Am J Cardiol 1985;55(11):1328–1331.

119. Deal BJ, Miller SM, Scagliotti D, et al. Ventricular tachycardia in a young population without overt heart disease. Circulation 1986;73(6):1111–1118.

120. Wren C. Ventricular arrhythmias. In: Wren C, Campbell RWF (ed): Paediatric Cardiac Arrhythmias. Oxford: Oxford University Press; 1996:127–156.

121. Noh CI, Gillette PC, Case CL, et al. Clinical and electrophysiological characteristics of ventricular tachycardia in children with normal hearts. Am Heart J 1990;120(6 Pt 1):1326–1333.

122. Vetter VL. Sudden death in infants, children, and adolescents. Review. Cardiovasc Clin 1985;15(3):301–313.

123. Case CL, Gillette PC. Treatment of ventricular arrhythmias in children without structural heart disease with class IC agents as guided by invasive electrophysiology. Am J Cardiol 1990;66(17):1265–1266.

124. Garson A Jr, Smith RT Jr, Moak JP, et al. Incessant ventricular tachycardia in infants: Myocardial hamartomas and surgical cure. J Am Coll Cardiol 1987;10(3):619–626.

125. Benito Bartolome F, Sanchez Fernandez-Bernal C, Jimenez Casso S. Incessant ventricular tachycardia and myocardial hamartomas in childhood: Long-term remission after surgical treatment. in Spanish.

Revista Espanola de Cardiologia 1997;50(3):205–207.

126. Kohli V, Mangru N, Pearse LA, et al. Radiofrequency ablation of ventricular tachycardia in an infant with cardiac tumors. Am Heart J 1996;132(1 Pt 1):198–200.

127. Villain E, Bonnet D, Kachaner J, et al. Incessant idiopathic ventricular tachycardia in infants. Review. in French. Arch Mal Coeur Vaiss 1990;83(5):665–671.

128. Zeigler VL, Gillette PC, Crawford FA Jr, et al. New approaches to treatment of incessant ventricular tachycardia in the very young. J Am Coll Cardiol 1990;16(3):681–685.

129. Fenrich AL Jr, Perry JC, Friedman RA. Flecainide and amiodarone: Combined therapy for refractory tachyarrhythmias in infancy. J Am Coll Cardiol 1995;25(5):1195–1198.

130. Batisse A, Sardet A, Fermont L, et al. Treatment of ventricular tachycardia in infancy and childhood with amiodarone. in French. Arch Mal Coeur Vaiss 1982;75(8):829–835.

131. Tsuji A, Nagashima M, Hasegawa S, et al. Long-term follow-up of idiopathic ventricular arrhythmias in otherwise normal children. Jpn Circ J 1995; 59(10):654–662.

132. Friedli B. Ventricular arrhythmias in children and adolescents. Pediatrician 1986;13(4):189–198.

133. Hernandez A, Strauss A, Kleiger RE, et al. Idiopathic paroxysmal ventricular tachycardia in infants and children. J Pediatrics 1975;86(2):182–188.

134. Hsieh IC, Yeh SJ, Wen MS, et al. Radiofrequency ablation for supraventricular and ventricular tach-

ycardia in young patients. Int J Cardiol 1996;54(1): 33–40.

135. Paul T, Trappe HJ, Pfitzner P, et al. Permanent ventricular tachycardia in a 12-year-old boy: Curative therapy by high frequency current ablation. in German. Zeitschrift fur Kardiologie 1996;85(8):603–610.

136. O'Connor BK, Case CL, Sokoloski MC, et al. Radiofrequency catheter ablation of right ventricular outflow tract tachycardia in children and adolescents. J Am Coll Cardiol 1996;27:869–874.

137. Wu JM, Young ML, Lue HC. An electrophysiologic study of a child with idiopathic sustained left ventricular tachycardia. Acta Paediatrica Sinica 1990; 31(6):360–365.

138. Suner S, Simon HK, Feit LR, et al. Child with idiopathic ventricular tachycardia of prolonged duration. Ann Emerg Med 1995;25(5):706–709.

139. von Bernuth G, Bernsau U, Hoffmann W, et al. Tachyarrhythmic syncope in children with structurally normal hearts with and without QT prolongation in the electrocardiogram. Eur J Pediatr 1982; 138:206–210.

140. Leenhardt A, Glaser E, Burgeura M, et al. Short-coupled variant of torsade de pointes: A new electrocardiographic entity in the spectrum of idiopathic ventricular tachyarrhythmias. Circulation 1994;89: 206–215.

141. Coumel P, Fidelle J, Lucet V, et al. Catecholamine-induced severe ventricular arrhythmias with Adams-Stokes syndrome in children: Report of four cases. Br Heart J 1978;40(suppl):28–37.

142. Leenhardt A, Lucet V, Denjoy I, et al. Catecholaminergic polymorphic ventricular tachycardia in

children: A seven-year follow-up of 21 patients. Circulation 1995;91:1512–1519.

143. Glikson M, Constantini N, Grafstein Y, et al. Familial bidirectional ventricular tachycardia. Eur Heart J 1991;12:741–745.

144. Cohen TJ, Liem LB, Hancock EW. Association of bidirectional ventricular tachycardia with familial sudden death syndrome. Am J Cardiol 1989;64(16): 1078–1079.

145. Dorian P, Strauss M, Cardella C, et al. Digoxin-cyclosporin interaction: Severe digitalis toxicity after cyclosporin treatment. Clinical and Investigative Medicine 1988;11(2):108–112.

146. Valent S, Kelly P. Images in clinical medicine. Digoxin-induced bidirectional ventricular tachycardia. N Engl J Med 1997;336(8):550.

147. Tsukada K, Akizuki S, Matsuoka Y, Irimajiri S. A case of aconitine poisoning accompanied by bidirectional ventricular tachycardia treated with lidocaine. Kokyu to Junkan—Respiration and Circulation 1992; 40(10):1003–1006.

148. Lucchesi BR, Chi L, Friedrichs GS, et al. Antiarrhythmic versus antifibrillatory actions: Inference from experimental studies. Review. Am J Cardiol 1993;72(16):25F–44F.

149. Trappe HJ, Fieguth HG, Klein H, et al. The importance of the underlying disease for outcome of patients with implanted automatic defibrillators. in German. Medizinische Klinik 1993;88(6):362–370.

150. Jordaens LJ, T Kindt H. Primary ventricular fibrillation: A reason to be cautious. Editorial. Eur Heart J 1997;18(6):890–892.

151. Tung RT, Shen WK, Hammill SC, et al. Idiopathic ventricular fibrillation in out-of-hospital cardiac arrest survivors. PACE 1994;17(8):1405–1412.
152. Wever EF, Hauer RN, Oomen A, et al. Unfavorable outcome in patients with primary electrical disease who survived an episode of ventricular fibrillation. Circulation 1993;88(3):1021–1029.
153. Peters S, Troster J, Hartwig CA, et al. Selective right ventricular angiography in apparently idiopathic ventricular fibrillation. Heart Vessels 1995;10(4): 211–213.
154. Aizawa Y, Naitoh N, Washizuka T, et al. Electrophysiological findings in idiopathic recurrent ventricular fibrillation: Special reference to mode of induction, drug testing, and long-term outcomes. PACE 1996;19(6):929–939.
155. Das G. Cardiovascular effects of cocaine abuse. Review. Int J Clin Pharmacol Ther Toxicol 1993; 31(11):521–528.
156. Willens HJ, Chakko SC, Kessler KM. Cardiovascular manifestations of cocaine abuse. A case of recurrent dilated cardiomyopathy. Review. Chest 1994; 106(2):594–600.
157. Anonymous. Increasing morbidity and mortality associated with abuse of methamphetamine—United States, 1991–1994. MMWR 1995;44(47):882–886.
158. Brady WJ Jr, Stremski E, Eljaiek L, et al. Freon inhalational abuse presenting with ventricular fibrillation. Am J Emerg Med 1994;12(5):533–536.
159. Adgey AA, Johnston PW, McMechan S. Sudden cardiac death and substance abuse. Resuscitation 1995;29(3):219–221.
160. Sato Y, Kato K, Hashimoto M, et al. Localized right ventricular structural abnormalities in patients with

idiopathic ventricular fibrillation: Magnetic resonance imaging study. Heart Vessels 1996;11(2):100–
103.

161. Raviele A. Implantable cardioverter-defibrillator
(ICD) indications in 1996: Have they changed? Am
J Cardiol 1996;78(5A):21–25.

162. Sweeney MO, Ruskin JN. Mortality benefits and the
implantable cardioverter-defibrillator. Review. Circulation 1994;89(4):1851–1858.

163. Meissner MD, Lehmann MH, Steinman RT, et al.
Ventricular fibrillation in patients without significant structural heart disease: A multicenter experience with implantable cardioverter-defibrillator
therapy. J Am Coll Cardiol 1993;21(6):1406–1412.

164. Nisam S, Mower MM, Thomas A, et al. Patient survival comparison in three generations of automatic
implantable cardioverter defibrillators: Review of
12 years, 25,000 patients. PACE 1993;16(1 Pt 2):
174–178.

165. Grimm W, Flores BT, Marchlinski FE. Shock occurrence and survival in 241 patients with implantable cardioverter-defibrillator therapy. Circulation
1993;87(6):1880–1888.

166. Belhassen B, Viskin S. Idiopathic ventricular tachycardia and fibrillation. Review. J Cardiovasc Electrophysiol 1993;4(3):356–368.

167. Shimizu W, Ohe T, Kurita T, et al. Effects of verapamil and propranolol on early afterdepolarizations
and ventricular arrhythmias induced by epineph-
rine in congenital long QT syndrome. J Am Coll
Cardiol 1995;26(5):1299–1309.

168. Crijns HJ, Wiesfeld AC, Posma JL, et al. Favourable
outcome in idiopathic ventricular fibrillation with
treatment aimed at prevention of high sympathetic

tone and suppression of inducible arrhythmias. Br Heart J 1995;74(4):408–412.

169. Quesada A, Sanchis J, Chorro FJ, et al. Changes in canine ventricular fibrillation threshold induced by verapamil, flecainide and bretylium. Eur Heart J 1993;14(5):712–716.

170. Nakazato Y, Nakata Y, Yasuda M, et al. Idiopathic ventricular fibrillation initiated by a short-coupled ventricular premature beat. Jpn Heart J 1996;37(2): 265–269.

171. Naccarella F. Malignant ventricular arrhythmias in patients with a right bundle-branch block and persistent ST segment elevation in V_1-V_3: A probable arrhythmogenic cardiomyopathy of the right ventricle. Review. in Italian. Giornale Italiano di Cardiologia 1993;23(12):1219–1222.

172. Miyanuma H, Sakurai M, Odaka H, et al. Two cases of idiopathic ventricular fibrillation with interesting electrocardiographic findings in Japanese. Kokyu to Junkan—Respiration Circulation 1993; 41(3):287–291.

173. Sumiyoshi M, Nakata Y, Hisaoka T, et al. A case of idiopathic ventricular fibrillation with incomplete right bundle branch block and persistent ST segment elevation. Jpn Heart J 1993;34(5):661–666.

174. Miyazaki T, Mitamura H, Miyoshi S, et al. Autonomic and antiarrhythmic drug modulation of ST segment elevation in patients with Brugada syndrome. J Am Coll Cardiol 1996;27(5):1061–1070.

175. Nademanee K, Veerakul G, Nimmannit S, et al. Arrhythmogenic marker for the sudden unexplained death syndrome in Thai men. Circulation 1997;96: 2595–2600.

176. Toyoshima Y, Nirei T, Kasanuki H, et al. Characteristics of body surface mapping in the cases of idiopathic ventricular fibrillation. in Japanese. Jpn J Clin Med 1995;53(1):168–173.

177. Schmitt C, Barthel P, Schmidt G, et al. Ventricular fibrillation and silent myocardial ischemia in a patient without anatomic heart disease. in German. Deutsch Med Wochenschrift 1993;118(41):1480–1484.

178. Igarashi Y, Tamura Y, Suzuki K, et al. Coronary artery spasm is a major cause of sudden cardiac arrest in survivors without underlying heart disease. Cor Art Dis 1993;4(2):177–185.

179. Malfatto G, Beria G, Sala S, et al. Quantitative analysis of T wave abnormalities and their prognostic implications in the idiopathic long QT syndrome. J Am Coll Cardiol 1994;23(2):296–301.

180. Grogin HR, Scheinman M. Evaluation and management of patients with polymorphic ventricular tachycardia. Review. Cardiol Clin 1993;11(1):39–54.

181. Jackman WM, Friday KJ, Anderson JL. The long QT syndrome: A critical review, new clinical observations and a unifying hypothesis. Prog Cardiovasc Dis 1988;2:115–172.

182. Schwartz PJ. The long QT syndrome. Review. Curr Prob Cardiol 1997;22(6):297–351.

183. Garson A Jr, Dick MD, Fournier A, et al. The long QT syndrome in children. An international study of 287 patients. Circulation 1993;87(6):1866–1872.

184. Priori SG, Corr PB. Mechanisms underlying early and delayed afterdepolarizations induced by catecholamines. Am J Physiol 1990;258(6 Pt 2):H1796–H1805.

185. Malfatto G, Rosen MR, Foresti A, et al. Idiopathic long QT syndrome exacerbated by beta adrenergic blockade and responsive to left cardiac sympathetic denervation. Implications regarding electrophysiologic substrate and adrenergic modulation. J Cardiovasc Electrophysiol 1992;3:295–305.

186. Tsien RW, Giles W, Greengard P. Cyclic AMP mediates the effects of adrenaline on cardiac Purkinje fibres. Nature—New Biology 1972;240(101):181–183.

187. Arlock P, Katzung BG. Effects of sodium substitutes on transient inward current and tension in guinea-pig and ferret papillary muscle. J Physiol 1985;360:105–120.

188. Moss AJ, Zareba W, Benhorin J, et al. ECG T-wave patterns in genetically distinct forms of the hereditary long QT syndrome. Circulation 1995;92(10):2929–2934.

189. Wang Q, Shen J, Splawski I, et al. SCN5A mutations associated with an inherited cardiac arrhythmia, long QT syndrome. Cell 1995;80(5):805–811.

190. Curran ME, Splawski I, Timothy KW, et al. A molecular basis for cardiac arrhythmia: HERG mutations cause long QT syndrome. Cell 1995;80(5):795–803.

191. Le Marec H, Schott JJ. Congenital long QT syndromes. in French. Arch Mal Coeur Vaiss 1997;90 (Spec No 3):25–35.

192. Schwartz PJ. The idiopathic long Q-T syndrome. Ann Intern Med 1983;99(4):561–562.

193. Schwartz PJ. The long QT syndrome. In: Wren C, Campbell RWF (ed): Paediatric Cardiac Arrhythmias. Oxford: Oxford Medical Publications; 1996:157–173.

194. Moss AJ, Liu JE, Gottlieb S, et al. Efficacy of permanent pacing in the management of high risk patients with long QT syndrome. Circulation 1991;84: 1526–1529.
195. Schwartz PJ, Locati E. The idiopathic long QT syndrome: Pathogenetic mechanisms and therapy. Eur Heart J 1985;6 (suppl D):103–114.
196. Kawade M, Ohe T, Kamiya T. Provocative testing and drug response in a patient with the long QT syndrome. Br Heart J 1995;74(1):67–70.
197. Noh CI, Song JY, Kim HS, et al. Ventricular tachycardia and exercise related syncope in children with structurally normal hearts: Emphasis on repolarisation abnormality. Br Heart J 1995;73(6): 544–547.
198. Sato T, Hata Y, Yamamoto M, et al. Early afterdepolarization abolished by potassium channel opener in a patient with idiopathic long QT syndrome. J Cardiovasc Electrophysiol 1995;6(4):279–282.
199. Bricker JT, Garson A Jr, Gillette PC. A family history of seizures associated with sudden cardiac deaths. Am J Dis Child 1984;138(9):866–868.
200. James TN. Long reflections on the QT interval: The sixth annual Gordon K. Moe Lecture Review. J Cardiovasc Electrophysiol 1996;7(8):738–759.
201. Oka H, Mochio S, Sato H, et al. Prolongation of QTc interval in patients with Parkinson's disease. Eur Neurol 1997;37(3):186–189.
202. Mohamed R, Forsey PR, Davies MK, et al. Effect of liver transplantation on QT interval prolongation and autonomic dysfunction in end-stage liver disease. Hepatology 1996;23(5):1128–1134.

203. Harris JP, Kreipe RE, Rossbach CN. QT prolongation by isoproterenol in anorexia nervosa. J Adolesc Health 1993;14(5):390–393.

204. Scott JL, Walls RM. QT interval prolongation. J Emerg Med 1985;3(3):221–225.

205. Metzger E, Friedman R. Prolongation of the corrected QT and torsades de pointes cardiac arrhythmia associated with intravenous haloperidol in the medically ill. J Clin Psychopharm 1993;13(2):128–132.

206. Zimmermann M, Duruz H, Guinand O, et al. Torsades de pointes after treatment with terfenadine and ketoconazole. Eur Heart J 1992;13(7):1002–1003.

207. Makkar RR, Fromm BS, Steinman RT, et al. Female gender as a risk factor for torsades de pointes associated with cardiovascular drugs. JAMA 1993;270(21):2590–2597.

208. Cowan JC, Bourke JP, Campbell RWF. Arrhythmogenic effects of antiarrhythmic drugs. Eur Heart J 1987;8:133–136.

209. Pye M, Quinn AC, Cobbe SM. QT interval dispersion: A non-invasive marker of susceptibility to arrhythmia in patients with sustained ventricular arrhythmias? Br Heart J 1994;71(6):511–514.

210. El-Sherif N. Early afterdepolarizations and arrhythmogenesis. Experimental and clinical aspects. Arch Mal Coeur Vaiss 1991;84(2):227–234.

211. Fauchier JP, Fauchier L, Babuty D, et al. Drug-induced ventricular tachycardia. Review. in French. Arch Mal Coeur Vaiss 1993;86(5 suppl):757–767.

212a. Thomas SH. Drugs, QT interval abnormalities and ventricular arrhythmias. Review. Adverse Drug

Reactions and Toxicological Reviews 1994;13(2): 77–102.

212b. Doig JC. Drug-induced cardiac arrhythmias: Incidence, prevention and management. Drug Safety 1997;17(4):265–275.

213. Wever EF, Hauer RN, van Capelle FL, et al. Randomized study of implantable defibrillator as first-choice therapy versus conventional strategy in postinfarct sudden death survivors. Circulation 1995;91(8):2195–2203.

214. Wyse DG, Morganroth J, Ledingham R, et al. New insights into the definition and meaning of proarrhythmia during initiation of antiarrhythmic drug therapy from the Cardiac Arrhythmia Suppression Trial and its pilot study. The CAST and CAPS Investigators. J Am Coll Cardiol 1994;23(5):1130–1140.

215. Ranger S, Nattel S. Determinants and mechanisms of flecainide-induced promotion of ventricular tachycardia in anesthetized dogs. Circulation 1995; 92(5):1300–1311.

216. Duff HJ, Stemler M, Thannhauser T, et al. Proarrhythmia of a class Ic drug: Suppression by combination with a drug prolonging repolarization in the dog late after infarction. J Pharmacol Exp Ther 1995;274(1):508–515.

217. Haverkamp W, Wichter T, Chen X, et al. The proarrhythmic effects of anti-arrhythmia agents. Review. in German. Zeitschrift fur Kardiologie 1994; 83(suppl 5):75–85.

218. Lazzara R. Antiarrhythmic drugs and torsade de pointes. Review. Eur Heart J 1993;14(suppl H):88–92.

219. Roden DM, Woosley RL, Primm RK. Incidence and clinical features of the quinidine-associated long QT syndrome: Implications for patient care. Am Heart J 1986;111(6):1088–1093.
220. Okada Y, Ogawa S, Sadanaga T, et al. Assessment of reverse use-dependent blocking actions of class III antiarrhythmic drugs by 24-hour Holter electrocardiography. J Am Coll Cardiol 1996;27(1):84–89.
221. Reisinger J, Shenasa M, Lubinski A, et al. Clinical implications of pleomorphic ventricular tachycardias on oral sotalol therapy. Eur Heart J 1995;16(3): 377–382.
222. Kuhlkamp V, Mermi J, Mewis C, et al. Long-term efficacy of d/l sotalol in patients with sustained ventricular tachycardia refractory to class I antiarrhythmic drugs. Eur Heart J 1995;16(11):1625–1631.
223. Morgan JM, Lopes A, Rowland E. Sudden cardiac death while taking amiodarone therapy: The role of abnormal repolarization. Eur Heart J 1991;12(10): 1144–1147.
224. Hohnloser SH, Klingenheben T, Singh BN. Amiodarone-associated proarrhythmic effects. A review with special reference to torsade de pointes tachycardia. Review. Ann Intern Med 1994;121(7):529–535.
225. Leroy G, Haiat R, Barthelemy M, et al. Torsade de pointes during loading with amiodarone. Eur Heart J 1987;8(5):541–543.
226. van de Loo A, Klingenheben T, Hohnloser SH. Amiodarone therapy after sotalol-induced torsade de pointes: Prolonged QT interval and QT dispersion in differentiation of pro-arrhythmic effects. in German. Zeitschrift fur Kardiologie 1994;83(12): 887–890.

227. Bashir Y, Thomsen PE, Kingma JH, et al. Electrophysiologic profile and efficacy of intravenous dofetilide (UK-68,798), a new class III antiarrhythmic drug, in patients with sustained monomorphic ventricular tachycardia. Dofetilide Arrhythmia Study Group. Am J Cardiol 1995;76(14):1040–1044.

228. Mattioni TA, Zheutlin TA, Sarmiento JJ, et al. Amiodarone in patients with previous drug-mediated torsade de pointes. Long-term safety and efficacy. Ann Intern Med 1989;111(7):574–580.

229. Siscovick DS, Raghunathan TE, Rautaharju P, et al. Clinically silent electrocardiographic abnormalities and risk of primary cardiac arrest among hypertensive patients. Circulation 1996;94(6):1329–1333.

230. Le Grand B, Hatem S, Le Heuzey JY, et al. Pro-arrhythmic effect of nicorandil in isolated rabbit atria and its suppression by tolbutamide and quinidine. Eur J Pharmacol 1992;229(1):91–96.

231. Rowland E. Safety profile of an antianginal agent with potassium channel operating activity: An overview. Eur Heart J 1993;14(suppl B):48–52.

232. Kempsford RD, Hawgood BJ. Assessment of the antiarrhythmic activity of nicorandil during myocardial ischemia and reperfusion. Eur J Pharmacol 1989;163(1):61–68.

233. Edvardsson N, Olsson SB. Induction of delayed repolarization during chronic beta-receptor blockade. Eur Heart J 1985;6(suppl D):163–169.

234. Fung AY, Kerr CR, Maybee TK. QT prolongation and torsades de pointes: The sole manifestation of coronary artery disease. Int J Cardiol 1985;7(1):63–66.

235. Kennelly BM. Comparison of lidoflazine and quindine in prophylactic treatment of arrhythmias. Br Heart J 1977;39(5):540–546.
236. Grenadier E, Keidar S, Alpan G, et al. Prenylamine-induced ventricular tachycardia and syncope controlled by ventricular pacing. Br Heart J 1980;44(3): 330–334.
237. Connolly MJ, Astridge PS, White EG, et al. Torsades de pointes ventricular tachycardia and terodiline. Lancet 1991;338(8763):344–345.
238. Day CP, James OF, Butler TJ, et al. QT prolongation and sudden cardiac death in patients with alcoholic liver disease. Lancet 1993;341(8858):1423–1428.
239. Stramba-Badiale M, Nador F, Porta N, et al. QT interval prolongation and risk of life-threatening arrhythmias during toxoplasmosis prophylaxis with spiramycin in neonates. Am Heart J 1997;133(1): 108–111.
240. Mehta D, Warwick GL, Goldberg MJ. QT prolongation after ampicillin anaphylaxis. Br Heart J 1986; 55(3):308–310.
241. James MA, Culling W, Vann Jones J. Polymorphous ventricular tachycardia due to alpha-blockade. Int J Cardiol 1987;14(2):225–227.
242. Antzelevitch C, Sun ZQ, Zhang ZQ, et al. Cellular and ionic mechanisms underlying erythromycin-induced long QT intervals and torsade de pointes. J Am Coll Cardiol 1996;28(7):1836–1848.
243. Tschida SJ, Guay DR, Straka RJ, et al. QTc-interval prolongation associated with slow intravenous erythromycin lactobionate infusions in critically ill patients: A prospective evaluation and review of the literature. Review. Pharmacotherapy 1996; 16(4):663–674.

244. Johnson A, Giuffre RM, O'Malley K. ECG changes in pediatric patients on tricyclic antidepressants, desipramine, and imipramine. Can J Psychiat 1996; 41(2):102–106.
245. Alderton HR. Tricyclic medication in children and the QT interval: Case report and discussion. Review. Can J Psychiat 1995;40(6):325–329.
246. Aldariz AE, Romero H, Baroni M, et al. QT prolongation and torsade de pointes ventricular tachycardia produced by Ketanserin. PACE 1986;9(6 Pt 1): 836–841.
247. Baker B, Dorian P, Sandor P, et al. Electrocardiographic effects of fluoxetine and doxepin in patients with major depressive disorder. J Clin Psychopharmacol 1997;17(1):15–21.
248. Warner JP, Barnes TR, Henry JA. Electrocardiographic changes in patients receiving neuroleptic medication. Acta Psychiat Scand 1996;93(4):311–313.
249. Bran S, Murray WA, Hirsch IB, et al. Long QT syndrome during high-dose cisapride. Arch Intern Med 1995;155(7):765–768.
250. Williams PD, Cohen ML, Turn JA. Electrocardiographic effects of zatosetron and ondansetron, two 5HT3 receptor antagonists in anesthetised dogs. Drug Dev Res 1991;24:277–284.
251. Bertrand ME, LaBlanche JM, Tilmant PY, et al. Frequency of provoked coronary arterial spasm in 1089 consecutive patients undergoing coronary arteriography. Circulation 1982;65(7):1299–1306.
252. Lewin MB, Bryant RM, Fenrich AL, et al. Cisapride-induced long QT interval. J Pediatr 1996;128(2): 279–281.

253. Chuang FR, Jang SW, Lin JL, et al. QTc prolongation indicates a poor prognosis in patients with organophosphate poisoning. Am J Emerg Med 1996;14(5): 451–453.

254. Little RE, Kay GN, Cavender JB, et al. Torsade de pointes and T-U wave alternans associated with arsenic poisoning. PACE 1990;13(2):164–170.

Index